WHAT'S YOUR PLAN?

Manage Side Effects of Chemo & Other Cancer Treatments

More than 90 natural supplements currently used in integrative oncology to support patients on cancer treatments

EVIDENCED BASED

"What a brilliant and much needed book. Incredibly comprehensive and extensively researched. To research all that's in this book would be far too daunting an exercise for anyone going through cancer to get their head around or have the energy for. All the hard work has been done with this book."   *Meredith (Australia)*

"Good on you for finding a way to help the friends and family members of loved ones with cancer to feel like they can really contribute and make a difference throughout the process"   *Rhiannon (Netherlands)*

"A single, comprehensive source of information. The holistic approach of this book is positive and encouraging, empowering people with the knowledge to make a difference to the quality of their lives while on cancer treatment... it constantly encourages communication with your health care professional, ensuring you are well informed and guided on the best possible path"
Alex (Australia)

JILLIAN EXTON

i

First published in 2012 by Jillian Exton
www.managesideeffectsofchemo.com
Copyright ©2012 Jillian Exton

National Library of Australia ISBN: 978-0-9872758-2-0

Should your friend wish to have a copy of this book, we would very much
appreciate you sharing our website www.managesideeffectsofchemo.com
with them so they may purchase a copy.

Disclaimer

The information contained in this book is for informative purposes only, and is in no way intended as medical advice, as a substitute for medical counseling or as a treatment/cure for any disease or health condition, and nor should it be construed as such.

Cancer is a serious disease which needs to be treated by trained, licensed medical professionals. Always work with a qualified health professional before making any changes to your diet, prescription drug use, lifestyle, or exercise activities. When seeking holistic providers, please ensure they are legitimate, medically trained clinicians. Sadly, there are unscrupulous individuals who prey on vulnerable people and promise "natural" cures to cancer in a potion or lotion.

None of the natural supplements in this book claim to eradicate cancer. However, there is substantial potential benefit in their ability to improve quality of life for cancer patients undertaking cancer treatment as well as provide an anti-cancer role, potentially by inhibiting cancer cell growth or increasing apoptosis (spontaneous cancer cell death).

This website includes links to other sites. These third-party websites are not under our control. Each link is provided for your assistance only to save you time and energy. We are not:

- Endorsing the products, services or information available via any named websites; or
- Making any representation or warranty about the products, services or information available via any of the names websites; or
- Endorsing or making any representation or warranty about the owner or operator of any of the named websites.

Acknowledgments

This book would not have been possible without the encouragement of my husband, Bruce, who was constantly by my side during my cancer battle and tenderly helped me manage the treatment of side effects. It was through these challenging times that the seeds for this book were planted. A hearty thank you also to Paul Battle, my neighbour, who watered those seeds when he asked me along to a conference which presented the tools and knowledge for me to take the next steps in this process.

Words cannot express my joy when I found two experienced board-certified naturopathic medical doctors in the United States - Dr Zora DeGrandpre and Dr Shelly Smekens - both as passionate and committed as I to the need to broadcast this information far and wide among the cancer community.

I am grateful for their courage in joining me on this adventure, as I know there are many skeptics and adversaries of natural supplementation theories for cancer treatments out there in the global medical profession.

To the many family, friends and colleagues that have provided feedback and wonderful suggestions regarding content, book titles, editing and formatting of this book - a huge thank you. You have all been a source of boundless support!

Bonuses

There are a number of bonus documents that accompany the purchase of this book. Should you not receive them please contact us through www.managesideeffectsofchemo.com, provide a copy of your receipt and we will forward you all bonus documents/books.

TABLE OF CONTENTS

Why I wrote this book …

So you've heard the words: "You have cancer". Those three little words can be terrifying and confusing. All sorts of questions are likely to run through your thoughts now and in the months to come. Why me? How will I cope? How will my family cope? What can I do to help myself?

Perhaps you have started to read and research some areas like nutrition and complementary support treatments for your cancer - and perhaps all that information has left you even more confused, scared and uncertain about what to do.

Having ridden the cancer wave during 2010 where I experienced surgery, chemotherapy and radiation, I was constantly looking for natural ways to proactively manage the expected side effects of my treatment. I was hesitant to add more chemicals than absolutely necessary to my system. Discussions with my medical team on possible natural supplements always resulted in the need for clinical studies and evidence to enable us to make an informed decision. And so the seed for this book was planted ...

This book is designed to give you realistic and solid information that you can take with you when you see your healthcare professional. Everything in this book has been fully researched, documented and explained.

A primary purpose of this book is to empower you, the patient, and empower your loved ones and support team as you proceed through the complex process that is cancer. Don't let cancer define you. You *can* be the one to help define the process and you *can* control your own health and wellness. While hearing those words: "You have cancer" is a traumatic, painful and scary thing, there is so much you can do to empower yourself, your family and your circle of support to overcome cancer and to live your best possible life.

Section Overview:

Section 1: What is cancer, what are the treatments and how do they work?

The first section gives an overview of cancer, chemotherapy, radiation therapy and other therapies you may potentially face, what they are intended to do as well as some of the potential side effects.

Section 2: What can I do nutritionally to help endure my cancer treatment?

The second section discusses nutrition - how you can best provide for yourself the vitamins, minerals and nutrients to get - and keep - your body as strong and healthy as possible *and* to minimise the levels of any additional toxins in your body.

Section 3: What can I do holistically to help me through my cancer treatment?

The third section provides an overview of Mind Body Medicine, explaining what it is, the science behind it, and how it can help.

Section 4: How do I proactively manage my treatment side effects naturally?

The fourth section provides detailed information about the use of natural supplements that are currently being used in integrative cancer clinics, particularly in the US. This section overviews a variety of natural supplements you can use to recover from surgery and deal with some of the side effects of your chemotherapy and radiation therapy. You will also find guidelines on possible drug interactions between natural supplements and treatment drugs.

Appendix

Now that you are aware of how these wonderful natural products can make your cancer treatment more comfortable, the appendix offers tables of all the supplements presented by treatment phase or by A to Z. There are also guidelines on buying quality supplements and links to reputable companies where you can buy products online.

Call to Action

ACTION At points throughout this book, we have added some actions to help you make changes to your lifestyle/eating habits.

Where to start

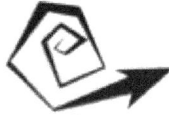

New to Cancer	Read **SECTION 1** to get an understanding of cancer, cancer types and the treatment approaches
How diet can support you through your treatment	Read **SECTION 2** to identify foods that may support treatment & recovery and what to avoid
How holistic healing methods can assist your journey	Read **SECTION 3** to appreciate how the mind can help your healing
How to manage your side effects with natural supplements	You **MUST** read **SECTION 4** to identify supplements to prevent & treat side effects. Then review the Drug Interactions table to ensure you will not impact the effectiveness of meds
Confirm your supplement strategy with your doctor	Read Suggestions on taking to your cancer specialist for tips
Where to purchase your supplements	Refer to **APPENDIX 4** for supplement buying guide and links to reputable websites.

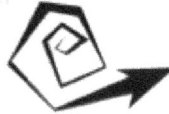

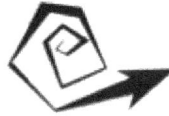

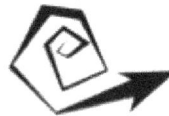

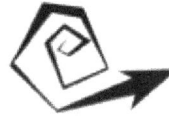

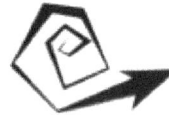

Suggestions for talking to your cancer specialist

Hopefully, you have found a cancer specialist you can be open with – and who is open to your questions, concerns and decisions. Many cancer specialists are concerned that natural approaches can potentially interfere with your treatment. Show them this book - we have made every attempt to document all information included here. You should remember, however, that your doctor and you make the decisions. We cannot provide medical advice because we don't know YOU! We can only provide information that is as up-to-date as possible. Use this book as an educational resource and discuss the information found in it with your doctor and all your health-care providers.

Finding an integrative oncology provider

This book offers solid, evidence-based approaches to supporting cancer patients before, during and after conventional treatments. However, it does not substitute for the recommendations, guidance and reinforcement of professionally trained clinicians. Please refer to the appendix for a guide to finding naturopathic physicians, holistic doctors, acupuncturists and registered dieticians.

> Use this book as an educational resource and discuss the information found in it with your doctor and all your health-care providers.

SECTION I: WHAT IS CANCER?

What is cancer?

All cells - at some point in their lifespan - have the capacity to reproduce. Our bodies contain many cells that reproduce by dividing into "daughter cells". Many types of blood cells, skin cells, cells in the digestive tract and sperm are examples of cells that are constantly dividing. The healthy body has control mechanisms to organise the methodical growth and repair of tissues. We need these cells to divide to provide for tissue repair, a healthy immune system, healthy blood and for fertility, and the control mechanisms generally do a very good job of directing this growth.

Our red blood cells have a lifespan of about four months. They carry oxygen to every other cell in the body, so we need to have them constantly replenished. Our immune systems are able to reproduce an army of cells which destroy damaging microbes such as bacteria, viruses, fungi and parasites.
In cancer, however, the control of growth and division of cells is disrupted and cells begin to replicate over and over again. This may result in a solid tumour or, in the case of a cancer of the blood, in tumours that may travel through blood vessels or the lymphatic system. (The lymphatic system helps drain excess fluid and helps removes various substances from your body.)

In general, while we often don't know the specific cause of any cancer, the DNA of individual cells becomes mutated or damaged and those control mechanisms for growth are also damaged. For example, a gene or gene group that helps control normal growth is damaged and the cells begin to proliferate (reproduce) rapidly and uncontrollably. Or, a gene which normally suppresses or inhibits growth can become mutated or damaged and no longer slows down the growth of cells. Also, during normal replication, the DNA must be copied; sometimes, during this process, mistakes are made and cancer may be one result.

Other mutations can create or act to wake up genes called oncogenes because of their involvement in growth. Oncogenes are bits of genetic information that can code for cancer. Most researchers believe it takes a combination or more than one mutation to cause cells to begin to grow out of control. But what can cause the mutation in the first place? Well, there are a number of factors to consider. First, the older we get, the more some cells have had to replicate - and it becomes more possible for a mistake or mutation to happen. Viruses are also known to cause cancer as well as substances known as carcinogens - cancer-causing substances.

Lifestyles may also put you at a higher risk for cancer. Smoking, excess alcohol, obesity, unprotected or unsafe sexual practices and a history of sunburns can increase your risk of specific cancers. Some cancers occur more commonly in families with a specific gene mutation.

Finally, and this is a big, wide risk factor, there may be environmental causes of cancer. This can include solvents that you may have been exposed to, air pollution, pesticides, herbicides, heavy metals and other substances such as benzene, formaldehyde and asbestos. This is often an area over which you may have little control and which we don't know as much as we'd like. Many, many different substances are released into our environment with little control and even less understanding of how these substances may affect human health.

An overview of the different types of cancer

We use one word, cancer, to describe more than 100 different diseases. Tumours can be benign (non-metastasising) or malignant. If they are malignant, there is a chance they may spread or metastasis.

There are a number of ways of classifying cancers, but the main categories are:

- **Leukemias:** These are a type of cancer that starts in blood-forming organs or tissues. Leukemias can be acute or chronic. Some examples are acute or chronic myelogenous leukemia, acute or chronic lymphocytic leukemia and hairy cell leukemia.
- **Lymphoma and myeloma:** These are cancers of the immune system. The lymphomas may be Hodgkin's or non-Hodgkin's lymphoma. Multiple myeloma is a cancer of the type of immune cell that normally makes antibodies.
- **Carcinomas**: These are cancers that arise from skin cells or from the thin tissues that wrap internal organs such as the stomach, intestines, breasts or the kidney.
- **Sarcomas:** These are cancers that arise from connective tissue or the bone. Connective tissue can include cartilage, muscle, fat, blood vessels, and other tissue. Bone cancer is also known as an osteosarcoma.

- **Central nervous system cancers:** These are cancers of the brain and spinal cord. Examples of these are glioblastomas and gliomas (astrocytomas).

There are some cancers that are gender specific - prostate cancer for men and ovarian cancer for women. Breast cancer is not gender specific - men can have breast cancer as well.

There are other cancers that tend to be more common in one gender or the other; for example, thyroid cancers tend to be more common in women while bladder cancer tends to be more common in men. We don't always know why, but it is thought that hormones can play a role.

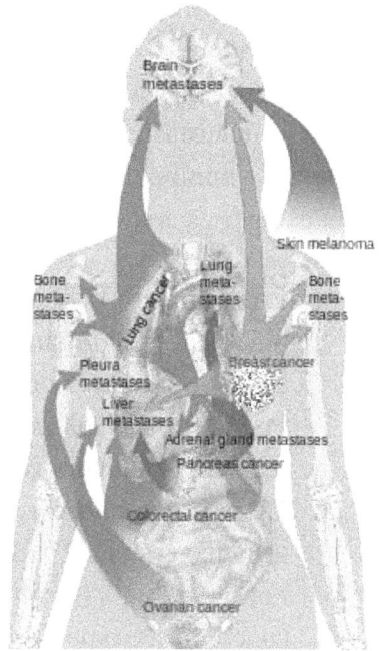

Cancer metastasis

Some cancers may metastasize, or spread, relatively quickly and easily, while others tend to spread more slowly. There are a number of routes for this spread.

- The tumour may grow into (invade) a neighbouring organ or tissue
- Tumour cells may break off the parent tumour and travel through the lymphatic system and the lymph nodes (lymphatic metastasis) or they may pass into the blood vessels (hematogeneous metastasis).

18

The most common parts of the body for the emergence of metastases are the lungs, liver, brain, and the bones.[1]

Most common symptoms of metastatic cancer

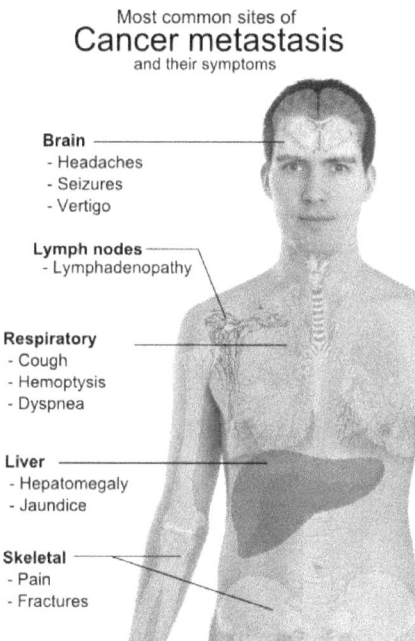

Most common sites of
Cancer metastasis
and their symptoms

Brain
- Headaches
- Seizures
- Vertigo

Lymph nodes
- Lymphadenopathy

Respiratory
- Cough
- Hemoptysis
- Dyspnea

Liver
- Hepatomegaly
- Jaundice

Skeletal
- Pain
- Fractures

Symptoms of cancer vary depending on the location, type and size of the tumour. Some of the symptoms of metastatic cancer are very much like the primary (original) cancer.

In general, the following symptoms indicate a need to see your health care provider.

Don't look at how you felt   yesterday when you compare; look at how you felt last week or last month. Keep a diary of how you are feeling; how food tastes, how much you are eating, how well you slept and so on. If you write down how you are feeling in a diary or a journal, it will allow you to better compare one week to the next.

- Fatigue that seems more than what you might expect;
- Any lumps or thickening on your skin, under your arms, around your neck or around your groin;

- Unintended weight changes - either an increase or decrease;
- Any changes in your skin such as a change in colour, redness, a yellowish tinge;
- Sores that take too long to heal or an increase in feeling sick;
- Changes in bowel or bladder habits that don't seem related to food or liquid intake;
- Constant or recurring indigestion or discomfort after eating;
- Constant or recurring muscle or joint pain that can't be related to your daily activities;
- A persistent cough;
- Difficulty in swallowing
- Hoarseness in speaking

An overview of conventional treatment approaches

Surgery

Surgery is one of the most common treatment approaches for cancer. If you have a solid tumour, the surgeon will remove as much of that tumour as possible.

Other areas such as lymph nodes and surrounding tissue may be sampled in order to determine if the cancer has spread and to gain a more specific idea of staging (a measure of how advanced the cancer is) and possibly the specific type of cancer, if that has not already been determined. Surgery may also involve the placement of a catheter or tube for the administration of chemotherapy or for blood draws.

Reconstructive or plastic surgery may also be done to recreate a breast or perform a bone graft, for example.

Chemotherapy

Chemotherapy (chemo) is the use of anti-neoplastic (anti-cancer) or cytotoxic (cell killing) drugs, either orally or by IV (intravenous, through the veins). There are many, many chemotherapeutic drugs, some used during part of the therapy only, some used specifically for one kind of tumour and some used for a variety of tumours. For our purposes, the most important factor is how and why they can kill cancer cells and how and why they cause adverse side effects.

Most chemotherapeutic drugs work by killing cells that are dividing - that is, by stopping mitotic cell division. Remember that cancer is the uncontrolled growth of cells, so chemo targets cells that are rapidly dividing. But other cells in your body divide as well. Some of the normal cells that rapidly reproduce are cells of the blood, cells of hair follicles, cells lining your gut, your mouth and your stomach. This is the reason - for a majority of side effects - those normal cells are being killed off as well.

Radiation Therapy

In radiation therapy, high-energy beams are delivered to the tumour. X-rays, gamma rays and other charged particles are most often used. The hope is to limit the exposure of healthy tissue by directly targeting the tumour and by protecting normal tissue. There are two main types of radiation therapy - externally delivered radiation and brachytherapy, where the high energy beam is delivered by placing a radiation source directly into a solid tumour. In either case, the radiation

21

destroys the tumour cell's DNA and thus its ability to grow. Radiation therapy is often done before, during or after surgery or chemotherapy.

Proton Beam Therapy

Proton beam therapy uses a positively charged particle - a proton - to deliver the radiation. There are two main types of proton beam therapy: brachytherapy, which uses radioactive pellet; and external beam therapy. The real advantage of proton therapy is that the treated area drops off quickly, reducing damage to healthy tissues in small spaces such as the prostate, near the eyes or in children who have smaller anatomy.

Brachytherapy

Brachytherapy can be either high or low dose. In brachytherapy, radioactive pellets or "seeds" about the size of a grain of rice are placed directly into the tumour. The low dose "seeds" are permanent, but because of the type of radiation used, they lose their radioactivity after a relatively short period of time. In the high dose brachytherapy, the "seeds" are removed.

External Beam Therapy

External beam therapy is also known as IMRT (Intensity Modulated Radiation Therapy)[2] uses other imaging techniques such as an MRI, PET or a CT scan to guide the radiation to the tumour. This is often done from many different angles. The intensity and the shape of the radiation beam can be controlled to give the greatest radiation to the tumour while minimising exposure to the healthy tissue. These treatments are most commonly delivered for about 10-20 minutes daily over a period of six to eight weeks.

Biological Therapies

Biological therapies use substances derived from biological processes as opposed to chemically synthesised drugs. This therapy is sometimes known as Biological Response Modifier Therapy (BRMT). Biological therapy helps your own body fight off the cancer cells, where in chemotherapy, the drugs kill the cancer cells directly.
Biological therapies include growth factors, vaccines and monoclonal antibodies. Therapy with monoclonal antibodies such as rituximab or herceptin may also be called targeted therapy because the antibodies are designed to "target" the cancer. Biological therapies include the use of BCG (Bacillus Calmette-Guérin), IL-2 (Interleukin 2) and IFN-alpha (Interferon alpha).

Angiogenisis Inhibitors

All cells need a blood supply to survive, reproduce and spread. Angiogenisis inhibitors starve the tumour by preventing the growth of new blood vessels to the tumour. Examples of angiogenesis inhibitors include bevacizumab, sorafenib, everolimuse and pazopanib.

Laser Therapy

Laser is actually an acronym for "Light Amplification by Stimulated Emission of Radiation) and comprises a single high intensity beam of light that can be directed at a tumour. Lasers are most commonly used to treat tumours on the skin, cervix and certain lung tumours.

Hyperthermia

Hyperthermia, or high temperature treatment of tumours, is most often used in conjunction with other therapies. In a hyperthermia treatment, the temperature of the tumour is brought up to around 111° F.

Hyperthermic treatment may, for example, be applied locally, to a skin tumour; regionally, to the abdomen, uterus or lungs; or to the whole body.

Bone Marrow & Peripheral Blood Stem Cell Transplants

The bone marrow is a primary source of stem cells - the stem cells divide to form new blood cells. Stem cells can also be found in the blood vessels outside the bone marrow. Both of these sources of stem cells can be used to "restock" your blood after chemotherapy or radiation therapy. Often, your own stem cells are harvested before the chemo or radiation therapy. This is an autologous transplant. For some patients, a bone marrow donor must be found - someone whose blood cells very closely match the patient's blood. These transplants are most commonly done to treat leukemias and lymphomas.

SECTION II: NUTRITION DURING CANCER TREATMENT & RECOVERY

One old saying you may have heard is "You are what you eat". Well, in real terms, that is very true. We digest the foods we eat and then use those digestion products as the bricks, mortar, siding, plumbing and electrical systems for our growth, health and protection. So, those leafy green vegetables you eat today will be helping to restore your bones, muscles, immune system and overall health tomorrow!

Cancer begins at the cellular level, where nutrition wields its greatest effect. Our nutritional status either weakens us, making us vulnerable to the development of cancer, or strengthens our bodies' defense mechanisms, enhancing our ability to protect against disease, fight cancer and avoid recurrence.

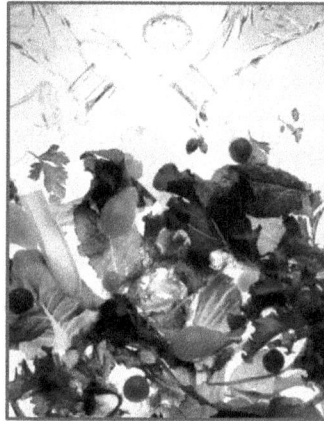

So an understanding of how we can use nutrition to best support our cancer treatment and recovery is essential. Our bodies are made up of and/or require:

♦ **Water** - there's loads of varying advice on how much pure water to drink, but a reasonable rule of thumb is 2- 2.5 litres per day. [3]

♦ **Proteins** - long chains of amino acids. Essential amino acids are required in the diet because our bodies cannot synthesise them. A "complete protein" contains all the essential amino acids. Proteins can be considered the "workhorses" of the cell. They are the main component of enzymes, substances that are essential to performing the hundreds of biochemical reactions that occur 24 hours a day, seven days a week.
Other proteins in the muscles for example, provide scaffolding for the cells and allow for movement. And other proteins function as signaling molecules, as antibodies in the immune response and a host of other functions. Proteins are also the primary component of our vital organs, muscles, skin, hair and nails.

♦ **Carbohydrates** - chains of various types of sugars. Carbohydrates can be complex chains of an assortment

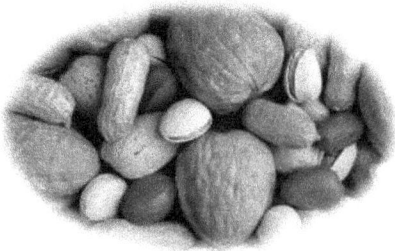

of sugars as you would find in, for example, whole grains or they can be simple sugars like the sugars you may add to your coffee ortea. Glucose is a simple sugar and so is fructose - the kind that is found in high fructose corn syrup. Glucose and fructose are both simple sugars, but their chemical structure is different.

The functions of carbohydrates are many and include the storage of energy, providing the backbone of DNA, RNA and enzymes, and providing structure to your cells. Fibre, necessary for healthy elimination, is primarily a carbohydrate.

♦ **Lipids** - lipids are a large class of substances and include the different types of cholesterol, essential fatty acids such as the Omega-3 fatty acids and triglycerides, among others. Lipids also can function as energy storage, structural elements of cells, vitamins and signaling substances.

♦ **Minerals** - We divide the required minerals into two groups: the "macrominerals" and the "trace minerals". Our bodies require quite a bit of the macrominerals and much less of the trace minerals. The macrominerals are calcium, sodium, potassium, magnesium, chlorine, phosphorus and sulfur. The trace minerals include, among others, iodine, copper, iron, manganese, selenium and zinc.

♦ **Vitamins** - vitamins can be divided into two main classes, the fat soluble vitamins such as vitamins A, D, E and K and the water soluble vitamins such as the B complex vitamins.

♦ **Intestinal bacteria** - the number of intestinal bacteria, by some estimates, is about 10 times the number of human cells![4] These organisms are essential for producing vitamin B_{12}, digestion and for certain aspects of our immune systems.

- **Other nutrients**. The list of "other nutrients" is long but includes anti-oxidants and bioflavonoids, saponins, phytoestrogens, organosulfurs and isothiocyanates. These are the types of nutrients you find in fruits, vegetables, tea and berries (anti-oxidants, bioflavonoids), vegetables (phytoestrogens, isothiocyanates (particularly in broccoli, cauliflower and brussel sprouts)) and whole grains (saponins). The organosulfurs are found in garlic, onions and chives.

- These are the nutrients that are so important for cancer prevention (especially the organosulfurs and the isothiocyanates) and for overall health.

What should you eat to promote your healing?

So, how can you get all these nutrients? Here are some general guidelines.

- Eat like your ancestors did! No, we are not suggesting you go off to some cave and cook over a campfire. But, your ancestors ate *whole* foods, not processed foods. They ate hormone-free game meat. They ate nuts, seeds, fruits and vegetables.

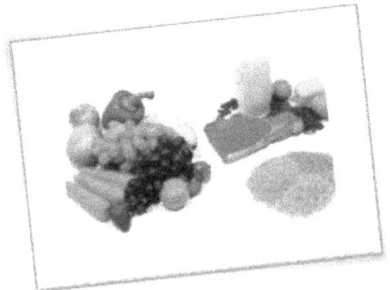

And the fact is our ancestors did not die from the same diseases we are prone to. Sure, the ancient Egyptians knew about cancer and heart disease - but most of our ancestors died of infections and injuries. The current epidemics are obesity[5,6], heart disease and diabetes.[7,8,9]

♦ Eat as many **fresh vegetables, fruits, whole grains, and legumes** as you can. Whole grains include brown rice, millet, oats, buckwheat, barley, quinoa, amaranth, corn, whole wheat, spelt, kamut and teff. Legumes are beans, peas and lentils. They include navy, adzuki, white, black, mung, garbanzo, pinto, lentils and split peas.
These foods are high in protein, complex carbohydrates, fibre, vitamins and minerals. They also help support the intestinal bacteria vital for digestive health.
Also be sure to eat seeds and nuts. The seeds can include sesame, pumpkin, flax and sunflower, to name a few. Head down to your local organic health foods store and check them out – try one new food a week and experiment!

♦ Try to minimise the fat in your diet, but keep in mind that some fats are essential to health. (See section on fats below.)

♦ Eat **fresh, whole foods** rather than processed, prepared foods. Processed foods may seem "easier" or more convenient, but beware the hidden costs. For example, during processing, many foods lose vitamins and minerals. Some may be added back; folic acid, for example is added into flours and grains. But, you may want to ask yourself, what *else* has been removed that hasn't been replaced? Also, many processed foods contain high levels of sugar, preservatives and other agents. The fact is we simply don't know what effect (or effects) most of these preservatives and other chemical have. They may be totally innocuous, but we simply don't know for certain. When you are trying to maintain or regain health, it seems prudent to remove any uncertainties that you can.

The term "whole foods" means grains and foods that have not had any of their components removed. Choose organic foods whenever possible; these will have fewer or no pesticides and other chemical residues on them.

♦ **Water, water, water**! Assuming healthy kidneys, the more water you drink the better hydrated you are and the better able to flush toxins out of your system.

♦ Increase the amounts of **nuts** and **seeds** in your diet - but careful of some of the roasted nuts and seeds as they may have been deep-fried or coated in oils and they may be overly salted.

♦ Increase the amount of deep sea **fish** and decrease the amount of meat - especially red meat - that you eat. Red meat in general has the wrong ratio of fats and is often filled with antibiotics and other chemicals. Wild caught fish is generally higher in Omega-3 fats than farmed fish and generally lower in various pollutants.[10] Some of the best fish to include in your diet are salmon, cod, trout, tuna, mackerel and ahi. Fresh salmon is an especially good source of healthy oil called eicosapentaenoic acid (EPA). Try to ensure that your fish is mercury free. Increase free-range poultry and eggs over red meats as well and avoid the skin. Avoid smoked meats that may contain nitrates or nitrites - these are nitrogen containing substances that have been associated with cancer.[11]

♦ Investigate the possibility that you have **food intolerances.** Gluten contained primarily in wheat products but also found in barley, rye and to some extent in oats, is one of the most common. Many people are also intolerant of dairy products. Some people are intolerant to both!

When an individual has these intolerance (sometimes called sensitivities), their digestive and immune systems begin to react against these foods, causing a variety of problems including digestive, neurological, autoimmune and musculoskeletal issues. Some people have discovered their sensitivities after years of suffering headaches, digestive problems, skin rashes, recurrent infections or respiratory problems.

When you are recovering from cancer or going through cancer treatments, it is reasonable to want to limit these types of issues, isn't it?

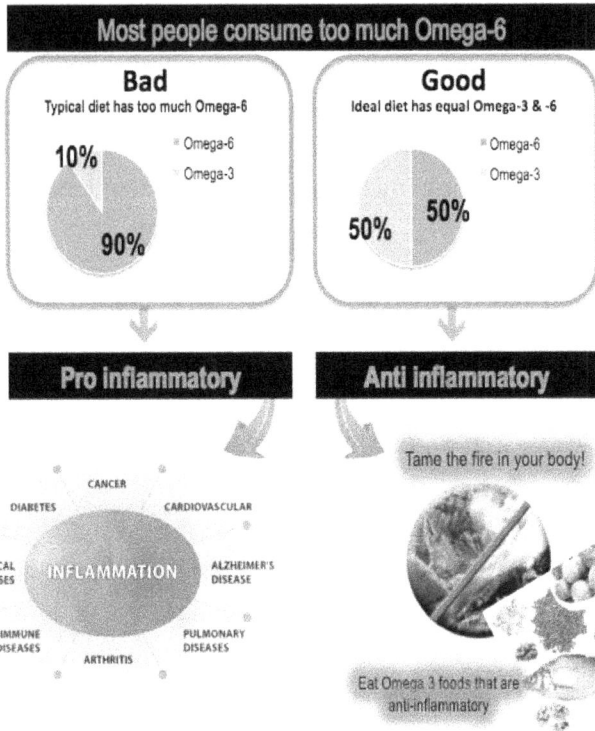

Most people consume too much Omega-6

Bad	Good
Typical diet has too much Omega-6	Ideal diet has equal Omega-3 & -6
Omega-6 10% / Omega-3 90%	Omega-6 50% / Omega-3 50%

Pro inflammatory → INFLAMMATION (CANCER, DIABETES, CARDIOVASCULAR, NEUROLOGICAL DISEASES, ALZHEIMER'S DISEASE, AUTOIMMUNE DISEASES, PULMONARY DISEASES, ARTHRITIS)

Anti inflammatory → Tame the fire in your body! Eat Omega 3 foods that are anti-inflammatory

♦ **Fats and oils**: Fats have been much maligned in the past, but the right fats are critical for health. Some fats - mainly Omega-6 fats - have pro-inflammatory functions, meaning these fats can support or increase the inflammatory process which in turn, can promote various types of cancer. Other fats - primarily the Omega-3 fats - are anti-inflammatory and subdue the inflammatory process. The issue lies in the *ratio* of Omega-3 and Omega-6 fatty acids – it's easy to consume Omega-6 fats because they are found in most vegetable oils. On the other hand, Omega-3 fats are found mainly in fish and in some plant sources[12,13] (flaxseed and flaxseed oil, canola oil, soybean oil, soybeans, walnuts, walnut oil, borage and purslane) and they are not as easy to obtain. So, people tend to have more Omega-6 than Omega-3 and *that* tips the balance toward inflammation. [14,15,16]

Our ancestors consumed about the same amount of Omega-3 and Omega-6 fats - a 1:1 ratio. We tend to consume more than 15 times more Omega-6 fats! In some countries, people consume 20 times more Omega-6 than Omega 3. Not too surprising given these are the same countries where inflammatory diseases are epidemic. In fact, while ancient humans died from trauma and infections, they did *not* die from chronic disease - every one of which is worsened or caused by inflammation![17]

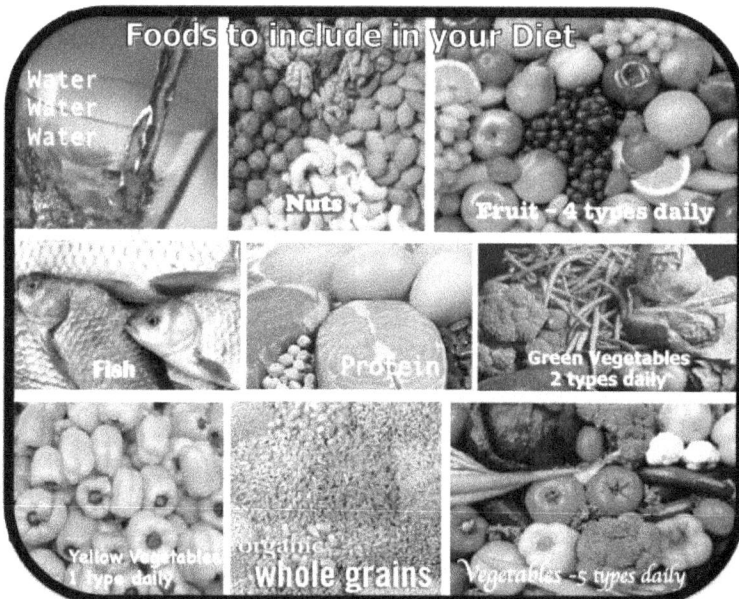

ACTION Change will not happen overnight; select one food from the section above to add to your diet this week. When you are comfortable living with that food, select another to add to your shopping list and experiment with in recipes.

Foods to Avoid

We've already mentioned some foods to avoid: processed foods, smoked meats, red meat and prepared foods. There are a few more foods to watch out for, though.

♦ **Sugary foods:** Most of us have a sweet tooth and no one is saying *never* have any sweet. But, highly sugared foods induce a rapid rise in blood sugar. That sets up a whole host of problems; the most recognised are increasing the risk of diabetes and heart disease, high cholesterol, insulin resistance and weight gain.[18] Breast cancer and colon cancer, for example, have been linked to obesity and inflammation. Fructose, particularly high fructose corn syrup, is considered by many to be central to an increased risk of obesity and moderation in its use is strongly recommended. [19, 20]

♦ **Stimulants:** This can be hard on people, but limiting the amounts of caffeine in coffee and black teas as well as soft drinks is advised. Caffeine can add stress to the adrenal glands and has been linked to cardiovascular disease and higher cholesterol levels.

- **Any foods with artificial colourings, flavourings and/or preservatives:** These products may increase inflammation and often their long-term effects are unknown.

- **Hydrogenated fats:** These are margarines and shortenings such as Crisco®. Instead, use pressed (or cold-pressed) vegetable oils such as corn, sunflower, sesame, coconut and canola oils, preferably in their unrefined form.

ACTION Change is an evolution; select one food from the list above to avoid this week. When you are comfortable living without that food, select another to drop off your list.

SECTION III: MIND BODY MEDICINE AND CANCER

What is Mind Body Medicine (MBM)?

In the US, the National Centre for Complementary and Alternative Medicine (www.nccam.nih.gov) is part of the National Institute of Health (NIH). NCCAM has defined Mind Body Medicine as a group of related yet distinct techniques thought to enhance the ability of an individual's mind - defined as thoughts, moods and visualisations - to directly affect their symptoms.

In Australia, MBM is similarly defined by Swinburne University, as focusing "particular therapeutic attention upon the role of the mind-body relationship in illness and health. The essential therapeutic aim is to promote bodily health and healing via the modality of mind - and through the mind-body relationship."[21]

MBM is a patient-centred approach, taking the patient's feelings, emotions, symptoms and needs, and working in a holistic manner and working to improve the patient's overall health and well-being. MBM places emphasis on the concept of healing past wounds and injuries, whether they are physical, mental, emotional or spiritual. MBM practitioners believe the mind has a largely untapped ability to surmount physical, mental and emotional limitations.

The term patient-centred is just that in MBM - the *patient* takes a central role in charge of their physical, mental and emotional self. The patient can choose to heal and seek recovery and they can approach their recovery as they choose. This empowering of the patient works with the various approaches and modalities and has shown clear cut benefits measured by survival and by quality of life.

An MBM treatment approach is considered successful - particularly in measurements of an individual patient's quality of life - if that cancer patient feels less depression and anxiety, is happier and more able to enjoy life. If that patient is able to laugh and play while enjoying the company of their family and friends that, too, is considered a success.

The main point of many of the approaches in MBM is that if an individual is at their physical, mental, emotional and spiritual "best", the treatments they have chosen are more likely to be successful.

Support groups, cognitive-behavioural therapy, meditation, prayer, positive visualisation, movement re-education, creative therapies, aromatherapy, yoga are all included as modalities of MBM. [22]

In a recent review of the literature in MBM, it was recognised that state of the mind—positive and negative – is of critical importance in how the patient responds to various therapies.[23]

Probably everyone is familiar with stories of how the mind and the mood can impact your health. Most people know at some level that the more depressed you are, the sicker you get.

We have also known for many years that certain personality "types" were more likely to

...other conditions - including cancer - that can be affected by how you think, feel and react to the various stressors...

have heart attacks - the business man with a "Type A" personality was considered at risk for a heart attack and told to cut back on his number of working hours and to get a hobby.

We now have much more evidence that it is not only heart attack but also other conditions - including cancer - that can be affected by how you think, feel and react to the various stressors in your life.

Another recent review connected the psychological, the nervous and the immune systems, with additional information about stress and the development of heart conditions, depression, various nervous conditions, hormonal imbalances, cancer and more.[24, 25, 26]

Humans have a physiological mechanism for dealing with short-term stress. But modern living has

In MBM, the effort is gathered around regaining and retaining the ability to deal positively and effectively with stress...

"stressed" the system to the point where it simply runs out of the ability to compensate for stress - and often, disease is one of the results. In MBM, the effort is centred around regaining and retaining the ability to deal positively and effectively with stress, and with enabling individuals to find peace and happiness whatever their situation is - and the result is healing and often cures.

A cancer patient undergoing cancer therapy has choices as well. You can see your cancer experience in a way that is positive, hopeful and helpful. You can focus on all the positive things that you may be experiencing - the help and support of family and friends. Perhaps now is the first time in a long time you can begin to care for yourself and your needs - there's nothing wrong with that!
Maybe you can do some of the things you've never felt you had time to do - even if it's as simple as watching the sunrise or sunset! Focusing on what you can do rather than what you can't may give you an opportunity to find out some of those things aren't really all that important after all.
Now just might be the best time to find out what you would *rather* be doing.

Is there any REAL scientific basis? Epgenetics

We've talked about diet, exercise, tai chi, yoga and relaxation techniques. Perhaps you are at the point where you are thinking this is all well and good, but is there any scientific basis and proof that these approaches are useful and helpful? The answer is yes. In fact, the answer appears to exist in our DNA and how it is monitored and controlled. The answer lies in a relatively new but rapidly expanding field called epigenetics.

Epigenetics is defined as the "heritable changes in gene expression that occur in the absence of alterations in DNA sequences"[27] "Epi" means "upon", "over" and "above", so it is a control mechanism over and above the genetic code - epigenetics is the study of the control of gene expression.

DNA codes for proteins-- and these proteins are central to continued health. Epigenetics studies how the DNA coding-- and therefore protein structure-- can be switched on or off by environmental and lifestyle factors - and the potential effects when a DNA segment (a gene) is turned on or off. When the genes are turned on or off, the proteins are either made or not made-- and this can seriously impact on a number of conditions, including cancer.

When it comes to cancer, there are a few important terms and concepts.

An oncogene, when switched on, can cause the changes necessary for cancer to develop but an activated oncogene can be silenced or switched off by a tumour suppressor gene.

However, if the oncogene is turned on and the tumour suppressor gene is switched off, the cells can become uncontrolled and cancer is a result.

Environment, stress, disease, mood and the food we eat can change our DNA in measurable ways - and these changes can be handed down to our children.

At its most simplistic, epigenetics investigates which factors can help turn oncogenes off and which can turn tumour suppressor genes on. And those turn out to be environmental, nutritional, emotional and stress-related factors.

It has been found that the environment, stress, disease, mood and the food we eat can change our DNA in measurable ways - and these changes can be handed down to our children.[28, 29,30]

There are hundreds of genes that are controlled using epigenetic means - these control the end results of stress, disease, the environment and food. And, this control mechanism is applied to genes important in the prevention and progression of cancer - the oncogenes and the tumour suppressor genes.

This means that our environment, the chemicals in our environment, our stress levels, moods and the food we eat can all affect our health, particularly regarding cancer. A number of genes known to be involved in the appearance and progression of cancers have been found to be directly affected by epigenetic changes.[31, 32, 33, 34] Some of these changes were related to environmental factors. [35,36] Other changes have been related to foods and dietary choices.[37, 38, 39] Still other changes reflect various lifestyle choices.[40, 41, 42]

Epigenetic research has also begun to focus on how epigenetics may be involved in how different cancers begin; [43] how some cancers can escape the surveillance of the immune system (which is thought to be important in destroying cancer cells); how it can be affected by the mind, by food, and by the environment[44]; and how these changes can then allow cancer to spread and come back. [45,46]

What is most critical to you as a cancer patient is the research showing that various factors - including environment[47, 48, 49], diet and nutrition, [50, 51] lifestyle choices [52, 53, 54] and emotional[55, 56, 57, 58, 59] - play a large and important role in the epigenetic control of cancer. In other words, it is becoming apparent that not only "you are what you eat" and "man does not live by bread alone", but we also are what we *think* and what we *feel*.

It has been said: "Technological advances make it feasible to envisage that in the future personalised drug treatment and dietary advice and possibly tailored food products can be used for promoting optimal health on an individual basis, in relation to genotype and lifestyle."[60]

Dr Dean Ornish and others [61] conducted a pilot study to examine changes in a group of men who had been diagnosed with prostate cancer and who for various reasons, had chosen not to use chemotherapy or radiation therapy. The gene expression in the prostate was studied after intensive nutritional and lifestyle interventions. The nutritional interventions included whole, organic foods and a balanced, nutritious diet. Lifestyle interventions included support groups, meditation, yoga and Tai Chi.

> When you add to this improved diet, lifestyle and an improved outlook, your chances of success can increase even more.

This study showed that after these dietary, lifestyle and MBM interventions, the genes changed. Even more stunning to the scientific world (and it *was* pretty stunning): this group showed that as the gene expression changed because of epigenetic mechanisms, there was a *significant* clinical improvement. 48 genes were switched on (up-regulated) and 453 genes were turned off (down-regulated). These researchers also saw significant improvements in weight, abdominal obesity, blood pressure, and lipid profiles.

The overall translation of this and other studies was that eating healthier foods, living a healthier life and communicating and sharing your emotional life with others resulted in an improvement *without* any drugs or surgery. This is not to suggest that you shouldn't consider chemotherapy, surgery or radiation therapy. That choice can be a life-saving choice - but it does indicate that when you add to this improved diet, lifestyle and an improved outlook, your chances of success can increase even more.

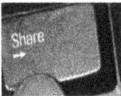

Wanting to share this book?
Email www.managesideeffectsofchemo.com to family & friends.

SECTION IV: NATURAL MEDICINE RECOMMENDATIONS

Introduction

The following recommendations are sourced from clinical research, animal research, in vitro data from laboratory studies of cells and traditional use. We have structured the natural medicine recommendations first by treatment phase: surgery, chemotherapy and radiation, then by side effect type such as constipation, fatigue, joint pain etc.

Drugs that potentially cause that side effect may be listed in the description. First look up your treatment phase; identify the side effect you want to manage and then review the list of natural supplements you can use to manage or support your treatment and healing. Please refer to the appendix section for a full list of all natural supplements by treatment phase/side effect and A-Z.

The Evidence Code

We have provided an "Evidence Code" that identifies the degree of research and evidence that exists to validate the use and benefit of the natural supplement to help you manage your side effects. This information will be important when talking with your health care professional.

- A. Clinical evidence in humans exists
- B. Evidence is based on animal studies
- C. In vitro evidence from observation made of cancer cells in a petri dish in laboratories

45

D. Historical data or traditional use validates the benefits

Please refer to the References Cited section in the appendix for links to abstracts of relevant studies, and related evidential studies. Be reassured that integrative medical doctors and naturopathic physicians currently use these natural agents to support their patients before, during and after cancer treatment. These recommendations are currently being used to decrease side effects, support immune health, for a direct anti-cancer benefit and, when available, to work co-operatively with conventional therapies.

There are natural substances that have been shown in research to make chemotherapy and radiation more effective. Natural medicine can also help before and after surgery to improve wound healing and recovery. The natural agents discussed in this book may have scientific names that may sound "unnatural" or manufactured but be assured that all of them are naturally occurring. Sometimes an extract or compound is derived from a fruit or herb to get to a higher potency of the active compound.

ACTION 1. Open the 'Natural Supplements to Manage Cancer Treatment Side Effects' excel spreadsheet, which you received as a bonus with this book (refer pg v 'Bonuses').
2. As you read through this section of the book use the filter and drop down list in the excel document to select the supplements relating to your cancer treatment and make a note in the comments section.

Buying a quality supplement

A natural medicine can work only when it is correctly cultivated, harvested and processed. When purchasing supplements, it is best to research the manufacturing processes of the company. All supplement ingredients need to be tested for purity and contamination, and all final products need to be tested for potency. Stability testing should also be performed to assure that potency is maintained at one and two years after manufacturing. This testing should be performed by an independent third party, not by the manufacturer and should be made available to consumers. This information is often included in paperwork distributed with the product, on the packaging of the supplement or on the website of the manufacturer.

Supplements should contain the correct/active part: for example, they should contain the root - if this is the active component - and not the stem or leaves. Herbal medicines and fish oils are especially susceptible to contamination from solvents used in extraction or from environmental pollution.

In the US, manufacturers should follow Current Good Manufacturing Practices (CGMPs) as described by the FDA (www.fda.gov). In Australia, the Therapeutic Goods Administration (www.tga.gov.au) regulates supplements and products. In the UK, it is the Medicines and Healthcare products Regulatory Agency (www.mhra.gov.uk). Check with these government agencies for manufacturers who adhere to quality control regulations.

In the appendix section of this book you can find a sample of professional supplement companies that adhere to Current

Good Manufacturing Practice Guidelines and a table with links to reputable online supplement companies where you can purchase supplements. Where possible, we have highlighted global health organisations or provided a link to different companies in Australia, USA and UK. Health food stores are good places to look locally for recommendations made in this book. However, be careful not to succumb to "armchair" medical advice from helpful store clerks.

It may be well intended, but these individuals are not trained medical professionals and do not know your complete health history or medication list. I can attest to this as a friend tried to purchase Vitamin B6 to treat his Palmar Plantar Erythrodystesia (PPE) – foot blisters from chemotherapy and the sales clerk talked him out of the purchase.

Feel welcome to take the information in this book to your provider to discuss therapies that can help you through your cancer diagnosis and treatment. Please recognise, though, that your doctor likely has no background in natural medicine and might be skeptical or outright refuse to let you take any substance that is not a pharmaceutical. Understandably given their training, many clinicians feel it is not safe to use natural therapies during cancer treatment.

Nothing could be further from the truth! Naturopathic physicians are working in hospitals in the United States and many other countries alongside medical oncologists to bring the best integrative care possible to cancer patients.

Drug interactions - safe use of natural supplements

Safe use of this information requires understanding the proper dosing and also knowledge of the possibility of negative interactions with your existing medications.

Drug interactions are unintended effects that can happen when two or more substances are consumed together: that is when one drug is taken in combination with another drug, or when a drug is taken along with a certain food, phytochemical, beverage or herb. Many drug interactions involve problems with the way the drug is absorbed, metabolised or eliminated from the body.

The Cytochrome P450 (CYP) system is a large and diverse group of enzymes in the body. The function of most CYP enzymes is to catalyse the oxidation of organic substances. CYPs are the major enzymes involved in drug metabolism, accounting for about 75 per cent of total metabolism. Most drugs undergo deactivation by CYPs, either directly or by facilitated excretion from the body. Also, many substances are bioactivated by CYPs to form their active compounds.

Drugs and natural substances are able to induce or inhibit the activity of CYP enzymes. Those that induce CYP enzymes encourage the body to make more enzymes available for action, sometimes reducing drug bioavailability by enhancing or accelerating drug clearance from the body and decreasing its concentration.

Drugs and natural substances that inhibit the activity of CYP enzymes may increase bioavailability by lessening drug metabolism and clearance, possibly resulting in extended drug effects and elevated or even toxic levels of that drug in the body.

Interestingly, some natural agents, such Curcumin, have been shown to increase therapeutic level without increasing toxicity.

The primary sites of interaction occurs in the liver and intestines where processing of many drugs and natural medicines occurs. You will find a CYP Drug Interaction table at the end of this section containing the most common chemotherapies, the enzymes involved in their metabolism and natural agents that can slow down or speed up this metabolism.

ACTION

If you are currently on chemotherapy medication, consult the table Chemotherapy Interactions with Natural Agents on page 106 before taking any supplements to check for any potential interactions. And please show this chart to your health care professional so they can help you make informed decisions regarding your supplementation.

SURGERY

Nutrients for wound healing

Surgery is a time when the body needs extra nutritional support to help repair tissues, support healthy immune function and decrease the likelihood of scar tissue formation. Fortunately there are nutrients from

KEY
A- Clinical Evidence in Humans
B- Animal Studies
C - In vitro evidence from observation made of cancer cells in a petri dish in a lab
D - Historical or traditional use

the natural world that can help your body recover from surgery.

Zinc: A mineral essential for wound healing, immune function and tissue repair. Zinc is required for the production of immune cells called neutrophils, natural killer cells, and T lymphocytes. Studies have shown that even mild zinc deficiency could negatively affect T-cell function.[62] Dose: 15 mg per day for 1 month following surgery.

Phase	Surgery		Side Effect	Healing
Evidence Code	A		Dose	15mg/day for 1 month post surgery

Vitamin C: Vitamin C is a cofactor needed for the formation of collagen and connective tissue. It is also essential for proper immune function. Following surgery, it is important to support the immune system to decrease the risk for infection. Vitamin C supplementation has been shown to reduce the incidence of organ failure and time in the Intensive Care Unit in post-surgical critically ill patients.[63] Dose: 1000mg three times daily for 1 month following surgery.

Phase	Surgery		Side Effect	Healing
Evidence Code	A		Dose	1000mg x 3 times daily for 1 month post surgery

Bioflavonoids: These nutrients are responsible for giving foods their vibrant colors. Bioflavonoids have anti-cancer properties but they also play an important role in blood vessel health. These colourful constituents improve the integrity and flexibility of capillaries, which are tiny blood vessels. After surgery, your blood vessels need to repair and perfuse the area where capillary structure has been disrupted. Several well-designed studies have shown flavonoids can accelerate healing of ulcers caused by venous stasis.[64] Dose: 200mg twice daily.

Phase	Surgery		Side Effect	Healing
Evidence Code	A		Dose	200mg twice daily

Bromelain: This nutrient has enzyme properties and is sourced from pineapple. Bromelain is strongly anti-inflammatory and helps decrease swelling following surgery. Its catabolic properties help to break up fibrin structures and decrease the formation of scar tissue. In a recent study examining bromelain use in colon biopsies, the nutrient decreased release of pro-inflammatory cytokines (molecules that act as messengers in the body).[65]
Dose: Take 500mg of bromelain two to three times daily for 3-4 weeks following surgery.

Phase	Surgery		Side Effect	Healing
Evidence Code	A		Dose	500mg 2-3times daily for 3-4 wks post surgery

Metastasis, or the spread of cancer

Modified Citrus Pectin (MCP) can help decrease the risk for cancer spread. Modified Citrus Pectin, also called Fractioned Citrus Pectin, is a naturally occurring polysaccharide that has demonstrated decreased rate of metastasis (cancer spread to distant sites) in animal studies. It comes from both the peel and the inside rinds of citrus fruits that is the white, it is the bitter pulp material that many people pick off and discard. Regular citrus pectin is not as easily absorbed into the blood stream as modified citrus pectin (MCP) as this form is broken into much shorter chains of polysaccharide.

MCP works as an anti-cancer agent in two ways.

- First, it decreases the adhesion or "sticking" of cancer cells to your body.
- Second, it inhibits something called the galectin-3, which is a mechanism the cancer cell uses to stay alive and not self-destruct.[66] Galectin-3 is more highly expressed earlier in the course of the disease, leading some practitioners to discontinue MCP after a patient has advanced disease and has been heavily treated.

The use of modified citrus pectin is not limited to one specific cancer type. A study in humans showed a substantial decrease in the rate of PSA (tumour marker) in men with prostate cancer.[67] A mouse model using implanted human melanoma tumours showed a dramatic 90 per cent decrease in lung metastasis.[68]

The recommended dosing based on the literature is to take 5 grams of the powder three times per day. If you purchase MCP in capsules, the dosing would be the same. Around surgery or biopsy, the risk for seeding cancer cells increases, which is why MCP is utilised to decrease the risk of spread. It should be used for 1 week prior to surgery and for one month afterwards. A patient is safe to take modified citrus pectin after they have returned to eating a full diet as it does need to be swallowed and digested.

The taste of modified citrus pectin can be quite bitter. It is a soluble fiber and dissolves easily in orange juice, yogurt or a smoothie. Reputable brands of modified citrus pectin include Allergy Research Group, Vital Nutrients, and Douglas Lab's Pectasol. There are no known limitations to taking MCP at the recommended dosing.

Phase	Surgery		Side Effect	Reducing the spread of cancer cells -metastasis
Evidence Code	AB		Dose	5mg x 3times daily for 1 wk prior & 1 mnth post surgery/biopsy

Decrease pain following surgery

Homeopathic Arnica: Arnica is a medicine derived from the wildflower *Arnica Montana* that has been used traditionally to help decrease pain, swelling and bruising following injury. The homeopathic preparation of Arnica does not have any interactions with other medications, so it is safe to take in combination with pain medications. There are two ways to dose homeopathic Arnica. Some practitioners recommended taking 2-3 pellets under the tongue as needed for pain. Others suggest taking 2-3 pellets three of four times daily in the weeks following surgery.

A study looking at homeopathic Arnica for pain management found it superior to placebo for patients recovering from tonsillectomy.[69] Patient undergoing elective face lift surgeries who took homeopathic Arnica had less bruising and swelling compared to those who did not receive the medicine.[70]

Phase	Surgery		Side Effect	Reducing pain, swelling and bruising
Evidence Code	A		Dose	2-3 pellets under tongue 3-4 times daily or as needed post surgery

Emotional support for surgery

Homeopathic Phosphorus has been used to help decrease the fear of surgery. Take 2-3 pellets of the 30c potency as needed prior to surgery to help decrease fearful thoughts.

Phase	Surgery		Side Effect	Emotional support
Evidence Code	D		Dose	2-3 pellets of 30c potency under tongue as needed prior to surgery

Homeopathic Gelsemium has been used to help decrease anxiety and trepidation regarding surgery. The dosing is the same as for the Phosphorus, 2-3 pellets as needed leading up to surgery.

Phase	Surgery		Side Effect	Emotional support
Evidence Code	D		Dose	2-3 pellets of 30c potency under tongue as needed prior to surgery

Rescue Remedy is a combination of flower essences to decrease nervousness and tension. It is available in a liquid, in pellets and in a spray or chewy. Follow the directions on the label to help with emotional distress and tension regarding your health and upcoming surgery. Bach Rescue Remedy worked better than placebo for controlling situational anxiety. [71]

Phase	Surgery		Side Effect	Emotional support
Evidence Code	D		Dose	Liquid, pellets or spray – follow directions on label

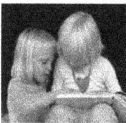

CHEMOTHERAPY

Cardiotoxicity (Heart) protection

The unfortunate side effect of some cancer treatments is cardiomyopathy or cardiotoxicity - put simply, damage to your heart. Pericarditis, inflammation of the membrane around the heart, can also occur secondary to cancer treatments. Cardiotoxicity occurs when the heart tissue is damaged and can take years or even decades to show up. Drugs that can cause cardiotoxicity include Adriamycin (Doxorubicin), Herceptin (Trastuzumab), Bortezomib (Velcade), Doxorubicine liposome (Doxil), and Mitomycin.

CoQ10 can help prevent cardiotoxicity. CoQ10 also helps alleviate fatigue, which is another common side effect of cancer treatments. Studies have shown that CoQ10 works by preventing some of the damage to the heart cells' mitochondria, an organelle within the cell that is responsible for energy production. An organelle is a structure within the cell that is important for proper functioning. Using a car as an analogy, the organelles would be the wheels, gas pedal and brakes. [72] Take 100mg twice daily.

Phase	Chemotherapy		Side Effect	Cardiotoxicity, fatigue
Evidence Code	A		Dose	100mg twice daily

L-carnitine: Studies have shown l-carnitine can help prevent cardiotoxicity and like CoQ10, it too helps combat fatigue. In an Austrian study, Non-Hodgkin's lymphoma patients taking L-carnitine showed no symptoms of cardiotoxicity from Doxorubicin.[73] Dose for cardiac protection is 500mg taken twice daily.

Phase	Chemotherapy		Side Effect	Cardiotoxicity, fatigue
Evidence Code	A		Dose	500mg twice daily

Note that L-Carnitine is <u>not</u> the same as Acetyl-L-Carnitine.

Taurine is an amino acid that helps regulates calcium movement in the heart muscle and acts as an antioxidant, scavenging free radicals. There are no good human studies showing cardioprotection from taurine used while on chemotherapy but there are several animal studies illustrating a definitive benefit. A Japanese study from 1988 infused taurine to rats given doxorubicin. The group of rats who got the taurine had increased overall survival and decreased blood markers of cardiac damage. Repeat studies have had similar findings.[74] The dose for cardioprotection ranges between 1000mg and 2000mg daily in divided doses.

Phase	Chemotherapy		Side Effect	Cardiotoxicity, fatigue
Evidence Code	B		Dose	1000-2000mg daily in divided doses

Constipation

Adequate hydration is essential for maintaining normal functioning bowels. If a person does not drink enough fluids, the stool can become harder and more difficult to pass. Even mild dehydration, called hypohydration can aggravate constipation.[75]

Phase	Chemotherapy		Side Effect	Constipation
Evidence Code	A		Dose	Gen health- drink 1/2 body weight in ounces /day. A 200-pound person should drink 100 ounces /day.

Magnesium Citrate: (A form of magnesium). Magnesium deficiency is common among cancer patients, particularly ovarian cancer patients, and is primarily due to poor intake, medications that lower magnesium such as Cisplatin and Alimta and loss through perspiration, diarrhea or vomiting. Symptoms of magnesium deficiency include constipation, muscle tension, weakness and cramps, difficulty sleeping and fatigue. The magnesium citrate form of magnesium works well to soften stools.[76] Dosage is 150mg to 300mg daily, higher doses should not be given without a blood test to determine magnesium levels.

Phase	Chemotherapy		Side Effect	Constipation
Evidence Code	A		Dose	150-300mg daily, higher doses

Higher doses should not be given without a blood test to determine magnesium levels

Probiotics are beneficial bacteria that live inside the digestive tract. They help regulate breakdown of food, appropriate secretion of immune cells and decrease the risk for overgrowth of pathogenic bacteria that can cause disease. Consuming healthy bacteria such as lactobacillus, bifidobacteria and saccharomyces boulardii can help regulate bowel movements, helping to improve both constipation and diarrhea.[77] Probiotics should not be taken if a person's white blood cell count falls below 2.5 as even beneficial bacteria can overgrow if there is a defect in the immune reaction to the bacteria. Chemotherapy can lower white blood cell count, so check with your doctor if you are unsure of your immune system status.

Phase	Chemotherapy		Side Effect	Constipation
Evidence Code	A		Dose	At least 5 billion cells daily

Probiotics should not be given when white blood cell count is below 2.5

Diarrhea

Chemotherapy, targeted immune therapies and radiation can all cause an increase in stool frequency and urgency. They can also change the consistency of stool so that bowel movements are too soft or even watery.

L-glutamine powder works to protect the cells of the digestive tract. Unfortunately, systemic chemotherapies can harm healthy cells in addition to killing cancer cells.   L-glutamine helps the digestive tract cells repair itself - from the mouth to the anus.[78]   L-glutamine also comes in capsules but it requires quite a few capsules to get to the therapeutic amount. The dosing for diarrhea is 10 grams daily. You can mix the L-glutamine in yogurt, water or juice.

Phase	Chemotherapy		Side Effect	Diarrhea
Evidence Code	A		Dose	10grams daily

Probiotics can help improve diarrhea as well as constipation. The beneficial microbes in your digestive tract influence the way your body digests and assimilates nutrients. Good bacteria also play a role in processing and removing toxins. Additionally, they contribute to proper formation of the mucosal barrier (the inner lining of the digestive tract), which is the gut's first line immune system. Lactobacillus acidophilus, bifidobacterium and saccharomyces boulardii (the latter is actually a beneficial yeast) are the strains with the most evidence for benefit.[79]   Purchase a supplement of at least 5 billion cells of probiotic bacteria for therapeutic benefit.[80]

Phase	Chemotherapy		Side Effect	Diarrhea
Evidence Code	A		Dose	At least 5 billion cells daily

Charcoal capsules. Activated charcoal is used in emergency medicine to bind with accidently ingested drugs or acetaminophen (Tylenol) overdose. It is utilised with chemo-induced diarrhea for similar reasons. The charcoal binds with the metabolised drug in the colon, aiding in excretion in the faeces. Irinotecan (CPT-11, Camptosar) is the drug where charcoal is most indicated, as the leftover drug is quite destructive as it passes through the colon, causing significant diarrhea in many people. A phase 2 study showed that activated charcoal with anti-diarrheal medications worked better to control Grade 3 and 4 diarrhea than the anti-diarrheal medication alone.[81]

Phase	Chemotherapy		Side Effect	Diarrhea
Evidence Code	A		Dose	Starting dose is 600mg 3 x daily, increase up to 2400mg 3 x daily

Fatigue

L-carnitine is an amino acid complex made by the body which works to shuttle fat acids into the cell's mitochondria, the organelle responsible for making energy. When the body is under stress or strain, it doesn't always make all of the required components of energy production. L-carnitine is made by the body from methionine and lysine and is found in animal products, tempeh (fermented soy) and avocado. L-carnitine improved sleep, mood and decreased fatigue in a study of cancer patients with advanced disease.[82] No adverse effects were reported and the most benefit was seen in the higher dose groups, up to 3 grams per day. The dose for fatigue is 1000mg taken three times daily with meals.

Phase	Chemotherapy		Side Effect	Fatigue
Evidence Code	A		Dose	1000mg x 3 times daily with meals

Note: L-Carnitine is not the same as Acetyl-L-Carnitine. Products containing L-carnitine cannot be marketed as "natural health products" in Canada. L-Carnitine products and supplements are not allowed to be imported into Canada (Health Canada).

B Vitamins are needed as co-factors in nearly every step of energy production. They help create ATP, which is the energy molecule used by the body's cells. Illness and taxing cancer treatments can deplete B Vitamins, which are water-soluble and generally not stored long-term in the body. The liver stores Vitamin B12, but it too can be rapidly depleted depending on need. Always take B vitamins with food as they

63

can cause nausea if taken on an empty stomach. B Vitamins have also been shown to improve feelings of wellness and general health.[83]

Phase	Chemotherapy		Side Effect	Fatigue
Evidence Code	A		Dose	1 capsule B complex daily or twice daily with meals

CoQ10, also called ubiquinol or ubiquinone, is an anti-oxidant and essential for proper energy production. Like L-carnitine it works within the mitochondria, the cell's powerhouse, but CoQ10 is also involved in the last part of energy production called the electron transport chain.[84] This nutrient is needed most in the heart, liver and kidney - organs that require a steady stream of energy to perform their functions. Dosing is 100-200mg daily. CoQ10 is not well absorbed so it's important to look for a product that is colloidal CoQ10 or CoQ10 in a lipid base (fat soluble) as this is the best absorbed.

Phase	Chemotherapy		Side Effect	Fatigue
Evidence Code	A		Dose	100-200mg daily

Rhodiola rosea is an herb that has been used historically for its benefits to stamina, mood and virility. Russian Olympians used Rhodiola to improve exercise tolerance. Rhodiola has been shown in research to improve memory, tolerance to stress and immune function. A double blind, placebo-controlled Swedish study found Rhodiola effective in treating stress-related fatigue, improving cortisol response, concentration and mental performance.[85] The dosing for rhodiola rosea is 100-

200mg in the morning and afternoon. Start with the 100mg dose. Taking rhodiola too late in the day can make it difficult for some people to fall asleep, as it can be stimulating.

Phase	Chemotherapy	Side Effect	Fatigue
Evidence Code	A	Dose	100-200mg morning & afternoon (start with 100mg)

Astragalus is an herb with anti-cancer benefit in addition to helping support immune function and decreasing fatigue. It is one of the most important herbs of traditional Chinese medicine, and has long been used in winter to ward off colds and flu. Non-small cell lung cancer patients reported a roughly 30 percent increased quality of life during chemotherapy treatment when given astragalus as compared to those receiving chemotherapy alone.[86] The only downside of astragalus is that you need quite a bit of herb to get to therapeutic benefit, the minimum dose being 3 grams per day and the ideal dose being 6-9 grams per day. Take 2 grams three times daily to combat cancer fatigue.

Phase	Chemotherapy	Side Effect	Fatigue
Evidence Code	A	Dose	2grams x 3 daily

Hand Foot Syndrome (PPE)

Hand foot syndrome (Palmar Planter Erythrodysthesia) is the redness, peeling and desquamation (skin cells sloughing off) of the hands and feet. It is very common with the oral chemotherapy drug capecitabine, whose trade name is Xeloda.

Vitamin B6 at 300mg per day works well to prevent PPE blistering (hand foot syndrome with Xeloda). If you can't find the 300mg capsules, then take 1 cap of 100mg three times daily. Take the B6 with food to avoid causing nausea. Women on capecitabine (Xeloda) for advanced breast cancer had lower than expected reported rates of palmar planter erythrodysthesia when taking Vitamin B6 or using urea lotion.[87]

Phase	Chemotherapy		Side Effect	PPE – (Hand & Foot Syndrome)
Evidence Code	A		Dose	300mg daily (or 3 x 100mg)

Use **antiperspirant deodorant** on the hands and feet to prevent the drug from seeping into the skin. It should be applied twice daily. Ban Roll-On is an anti-perspirant that doesn't have an odour. Tom's of Maine also makes an unscented anti-perspirant that is naturally derived.

Phase	Chemotherapy		Side Effect	PPE – (Hand & Foot Syndrome)
Evidence Code	A		Dose	Apply twice daily

Aggressive skin hydration: Use a natural lotion without harsh chemicals or preservatives to keep the hands and feet moistened. If liberal lotion use is not enough, apply a thick cream to the hands and feet at night and then wear cotton gloves and cotton socks to avoid getting the sheets greasy. Skin hydration will help prevent the cracking of the palms of the hands and soles of the feet that can occur with hand foot syndrome. Urea ointment has reported benefit with hand foot syndrome. (see study referenced above under Vitamin B6 recommendation.)

Phase	Chemotherapy	Side Effect	PPE – (Hand & Foot Syndrome)
Evidence Code	AD	Dose	Use liberally or thick cream at night

Henna has been shown effective in decreasing PPE, but it does discolour the hands and feet an orangey brown. This phenomenon was accidentally discovered; Turkish women reported having reduced symptoms of PPE when their hands and feet were decorated with Henna for wedding celebrations. A case series was published in 2008 showing that henna reduced, and even resolved in some individuals, grade 2 and grade 3 hand foot syndrome.[88] It was believed that these results were from the analgesic and anti-inflammatory effects of henna.

Phase	Chemotherapy	Side Effect	PPE – (Hand & Foot Syndrome)
Evidence Code	A	Dose	Topical application to affected areas

Topical DMSO, an anti-inflammatory sulphur compound has been shown to help alleviate the symptoms of hand foot syndrome from Xeloda. A compounding pharmacist can prepare a DMSO lotion of 99 per cent strength, which was the

67

concentration used four times daily in a 1999 study.[89] Creams and lotions of lesser strength can also have some benefit.

Phase	Chemotherapy
Evidence Code	A

Side Effect	PPE – (Hand & Foot Syndrome)
Dose	Use 4 x daily

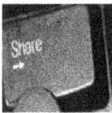

Hot flushes

Hormone blocking therapies are used to treat breast and prostate cancers. Common drugs used for this purpose in cancer patients include Tamoxifen, Anastrazole (Arimidex), Leuprolide (Lupron), Abarelix, Goserelin (Zoladex), Letrozole (Femara), and Exemestane (Aromasin).

Black Cohosh is an herb long used for menopausal symptoms hot flushes.[90] Its mechanism of action for reducing hot flushes is under debate. Some experts label this herb as estrogenic but there is research that it also exhibits anti-estrogen activity. Alcohol extracts of the root do not seem to have estrogenic activity yet it, too, has been reported to help alleviate hot flushes. Perhaps the phytosterols, vitamins, minerals and isoflavinoids also play a role in temperature regulation and blood vessel spasm. Black cohosh has been demonstrated to help alleviate hot flushes from cancer hormonal therapies. Black cohosh does not have an estrogenic affect on the breast.[91]

Phase	Chemotherapy
Evidence Code	A

Side Effect	Hot Flushes
Dose	80-100mg twice daily

Vitamin C strengthens blood vessels and is an active anti-oxidant. It has long been purported for anti-cancer benefits and immune system support. It has been suggested that in addition to supporting blood vessel health, Vitamin C may reduce hot flushes by providing support to the adrenal glands, which sit atop the kidneys and help regulate stress response, blood pressure, blood sugar and hormones. Since many hot flushes are triggered during times of stress, Vitamin C may help to modify the body's response to that stress by providing nutritional support to the adrenals.[92] Dose for hot flushes is 1000mg taken 3 times daily.

Phase	Chemotherapy		Side Effect	Hot Flushes
Evidence Code	A		Dose	1000mg 3 x daily

Hesperidin is a bioflavonoid that helps hot flushes by improving blood vessel health and integrity. Interestingly, hesperidin has also been studied for its anti-cancer benefits both as an anti-oxidant and as an angiogenesis inhibitor, which means that it discourages cancer cells from making new blood vessels. An early clinical study looking at nutritional interventions for hot flushes found the combination of hesperidin and Vitamin C used for one month eliminated hot flushes in 53 per cent of the subjects and reduced them in an additional 34 per cent of the women.[93] Starting dose is 250 mg taken 3 times daily.

Phase	Chemotherapy		Side Effect	Hot Flushes
Evidence Code	A		Dose	250mg 3 x daily

5-HTP is the precursor to serotonin, the neurotransmitter responsible for mood and made famous by commercials for the SSRI (selective serotonin reuptake inhibitors) anti-depressants. Beyond mood, serotonin is also involved in the hypothalamus' signals to the body to tell the blood vessels to dilate or constrict. The hypothalamus is a structure in your brain that links your nervous system to your endocrine (hormone)

70

system. Increasing serotonin is thought to work by adjusting the brain's thermoregulation (temperature regulation).[94] The recommended dose for hot flushes is 50-100mg three times daily.

Phase	Chemotherapy
Evidence Code	D

Side Effect	Hot Flushes
Dose	50-100mg 3 x daily

> *5-HTP should not be taken with SSRIs or MAOI without the supervision of a physician. MAOIs are antidepressant drugs and include Phenelzine (Nardil), isocarboxazid (Marplan) and Selegilene (Zelapar or Eldepryl)*

Soy isoflavones act as phytoestrogens, stimulating estrogen receptors but with a fraction of the power of regular estrogen hormones. Estrogens act on both serotonin receptors and the preoptic nucleus in the brain to change the normal temperature set point. There is some debate about the role of soy in breast cancer. Dietary intake of soy foods in observational studies has shown lower cancer rates among those eating and drinking soy.

It was theorised that once a person has breast cancer, the soy could stimulate estrogen receptor positive tumours or could lead to higher recurrence rates. Recently, large studies by Vanderbilt University have allayed much of this fear as they tracked women with breast cancer and those with a history of breast cancer. Breast cancer survivors did *not* have any difference in disease recurrence if they consumed 1 soy food or drink per day.[95]

71

Even more interestingly, a study of women in Shanghai with breast cancer had lower death rates and lower recurrence rate.[96] The use of soy supplements was not included in those studies. The authors stated that, *"Soy food consumption after cancer diagnosis, measured as soy protein intake, was inversely associated with mortality and recurrence."* The dose is 15-20 grams of soy protein or 50mg of soy isoflavones per day.

Phase	Chemotherapy	Side Effect	Hot Flushes
Evidence Code	A	Dose	12-20grams of soy protein or 50mg of soy isoflavones daily

Magnesium can help with hot flushes, speculated to work by decreasing vasospasm of blood vessels. A clinical trial of breast cancer patients showed magnesium worked to decrease hot flash symptoms in more than half of the women.[97] The low cost and high safety of this mineral make it a good choice for first line therapy in hot flash management. Dose in this recent study was 400mg daily, increased to 800mg daily if needed. Magnesium at this dosing should not be taken in patients with advanced kidney disease or electrolyte disturbance without a doctor's supervision.

Phase	Chemotherapy	Side Effect	Hot Flushes
Evidence Code	A	Dose	400 to 800mg daily in divided doses

Insomnia

Melatonin is a hormone produced by a tiny gland in the brain called the pineal gland. It is secreted mostly during the evening during sleep. Melatonin has also been studied for its anti-cancer benefits and antioxidant function. Dosage for sleep is 3 to 5 mg taken 30 minutes before desired bedtime. Dosage for anti-cancer benefit is 20mg before bed. In rare cases, melatonin can cause vivid dreaming or next-day fatigue but this is experienced in less than 5 per cent of people. Long term use of melatonin has been shown to improve sleep quality without adverse affects on development or mood.[98]

Phase	Chemotherapy		Side Effect	Insomnia
Evidence Code	A		Dose	1. Sleep-3-5mg 30 min before desired bed time 2. Anti Cancer- 20mg 30 min before desired bed time

Theanine is an amino acid molecule found in green tea that reduces stimulation of glutamate receptors in the brain, promoting relaxation and sleep. It has been discovered to reduce the death of neurons (nerve cells inside the brain) from overstimulation and oxidative stress. Researchers subjected human participants to rigorous mental tasks: when the subjects were given l-theanine prior to the difficult work, they had lower physiological stress response as compared to placebo.[99] The dosing for sleep is 100mg with dinner or before bed.

Phase	Chemotherapy		Side Effect	Insomnia
Evidence Code	A		Dose	100mg 30 with dinner or before bed

Inositol is a nutrient in the B vitamin family that is very calming. An Israeli clinical trial found inositol to work better than standard anti-depressants in reducing frequency of panic attacks.[100] It's useful for insomnia where anxiety is preventing sleep. Dosing is between 3 and 6 grams daily in divided doses for decreasing anxiety. Start with 3 grams daily and increase up to 6 grams as needed to help with anxiety. Specifically for use prior to bed, 1 gram should be taken 1 hour prior to bedtime.

Phase	Chemotherapy
Evidence Code	A

Side Effect	Insomnia
Dose	3-6grams daily & increase up to 6 grams. For sleep take 1 gram 1 hr prior to bed

Joint pain (Arthralgias) and general pain

Some cancer therapies, including hormonal treatments and targeted chemotherapeutics, can cause joint pain. This pain can be the result of inflammation, immune stimulation or bone loss. Drugs with arthralagia as a side effect include bleomycin, filgrastim, paclitaxel, and letrozole and L-asparaginase.

Unfortunately, pain is a common side effect of many cancers. There are many medications that can help relieve pain but they, too, come with a series of side effects including drowsiness, constipation and fatigue. There are some natural agents that are analgesic (can reduce pain) but they should never serve as a substitute for your medications if your pain is not controlled. Pain is not therapeutic and needs to be addressed with a plan from your physician(s). The following recommendations can help reduce pain and potentially your need for pain medications.

Bromelain is an enzyme found in pineapple that can help decrease inflammation, minimize scar tissue and alleviate pain. A study appearing in a German Rheumatology journal found a bromelain enzyme formula as effective as standard anti-inflammatory pain medication (NSAIDs - NonSteroidalAnti-InflammatoryDrugs such as Tylenol and Ibuprofen) in reducing hip pain.[101] Bromelain is also used post-surgery to help with wound healing.

Phase	Chemotherapy		Side Effect	Joint pain
Evidence Code	A		Dose	200mg twice daily

Glucosamine & Chondroitin: Glucosamine is a monosaccharide that serves as the building block for synthesising glycosaminoglycans, a material that is part of the cartilage of joints. Glucosamine can help decrease joint pain by restoring the cartilage, which serves as a sort of buffer zone between two bones. Glucosamine is often sold in combination with chondroitin, another glycosaminoglycan utilised in cartilage. Interestingly, a recent study found long term use of glucosamine, greater than 10 years, decreased risk of developing lung cancer.[102] Dosing is 1500mg of glucosamine and 1000mg of chondroitin daily.

Phase	Chemotherapy		Side Effect	Joint pain
Evidence Code	A		Dose	1500mg glucosamine and 1000mg chondroitin daily

MSM (Methylsulfonylmethane) is a sulphur-containing compound that is strongly anti-inflammatory. In the body, roughly 15 per cent of DMSO (another popular supplement) is changed into MSM. Sulphur rich DMSO and MSM have been shown to improve joint pain and muscle aches.[103] They have also been studied for benefit with interstitial cystitis (a urinary bladder disorder) and with seasonal allergies. In vitro, DMSO is a COX 2 inhibitor similar to the mechanism of action of NSAIDs - pharmaceutical anti-inflammatories. COX 2 (for CycloOxygenase-2) is an enzyme that causes inflammation and pain when provoked by a stimulus, such as an activated immune system. The dosing of MSM is 1000mg three times daily.

Phase	Chemotherapy		Side Effect	Joint pain
Evidence Code	A		Dose	1000mg x 3 times daily

Curcumin, extract comes from turmeric, a root used in Indian cooking that gives curry its characteristic yellow orange colour is an herb that can decrease inflammation and pain. It could be argued that curcumin's anti-cancer potential eclipses all other herbs. There are seven (and possibly more) different mechanisms by which curcumin has been shown to halt the progress of carcinogenesis.[104] A double blind, placebo-controlled post-surgical study showed curcumin decreased pain and fatigue following gall bladder removal.[105] Dosing for pain is 1000mg 3 to 4 times daily.

Phase	Chemotherapy		Side Effect	Joint pain
Evidence Code	A		Dose	1000mg x 3-4 times daily

Mucositis (Mouth sores)

Cancer patients undergoing chemotherapy for leukemia and lymphoma have some of the highest rates of mucositis, as do those patients receiving radiation to the head or neck. Chemotherapies that commonly have mouth sores as a side effect include bleomycin, doxorubicin, edatrexate, fluorouracil, methotrexate and topotecan.

Honey is anti-microbial, anti-inflammatory and can inhibit the growth of both fungus and bacteria. It also helps heal epithelial tissue, which comprises the outermost cells of the mouth. Studies show the anti-cancer benefit of honey in a variety of malignancies. Studies of Manuka honey have shown both a preventative and treatment role. An Egyptian clinical trial found honey effectively helped prevent mucositis in patients receiving chemotherapy and radiation for head and neck cancers.[106] Manuka honey is a variety made from New Zealand pollen that has the most published evidence for benefit.

Phase	Chemotherapy
Evidence Code	A

Side Effect	Mouth sores
Dose	1 tea -1 tablespoon applied to sore areas 3-4 times daily. Can also be added to food and eaten.

L-glutamine repairs cells of the digestive tract, including those inside the mouth. Put approximately 10 grams of l-glutamine into 4 ounces of water and swish inside your mouth. Alternatively, you can add a small amount of water to the l-glutamine powder and form a paste, which can be applied directly to the mouth sores. Research has shown glutamine to have benefit in preventing both radiation and chemotherapy induced mucositis.[107] [108]

Phase	Chemotherapy
Evidence Code	A

Side Effect	Mouth sores
Dose	10 grams in 4 ounces of water & rinse mouth OR make a paste and apply

DGL, the abbreviated name of deglycyrrhizinated licorice, is a form of licorice that promotes healing of the lining of the digestive tract. It's used for gastritis (stomach irritation), cold sores and acid reflux.[109] DGL is available in powder, liquid, capsules or chewable tablets. It's important the herb have contact with the mouth so if you purchase a capsule, it needs to be opened.

Phase	Chemotherapy
Evidence Code	AD

Side Effect	Mouth sores
Dose	Apply to mouth sores

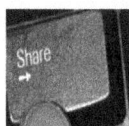

Neuropathy

Neuropathy is a disorder of nerves and can appear as symptoms of numbness, pain, burning and sensory loss caused by damage to the nerves. Diabetes and chemotherapy are the most common causes of neuropathy, and have their most pronounced effects on peripheral nerves, which affects the hands and feet. Early neuropathic changes can cause numbness, tingling or slight decreases in sensation. Advanced neuropathy can inhibit normal walking or grasping and can be excruciating painful.

The following recommendations can help heal existing neuropathy but really work best prophylactically - preventatively, that is *before* symptoms are present or are just beginning. Physical therapy can also be very useful in treating neuropathy. Both acupuncture and physiotherapy using electrical stimulation can be especially helpful.

Vitamin B6. This B vitamin is involved in more than 100 enzymatic reactions in the body. B6 is vital for proper immune function as it increases the manufacturing of immune cells called lymphocytes (white blood cells). Diabetic neuropathy has long been treated with B vitamins, including B6 but now research supports its use for chemotherapy-induced neuropathy as well. An Indian study of children treated with vincristine chemotherapy showed complete resolution of neuropathy with Vitamin B6 administration. [110] The dose required to prevent neuropathy is 300mg per day taken with food.

Phase	Chemotherapy		Side Effect	Neuropathy
Evidence Code	A		Dose	300mg daily with food

L-glutamine powder is useful for treating diarrhea and mucositis, but it is also beneficial for the prevention of neuropathy. Paclitaxel, a drug known for causing peripheral neuropathy, was given with or without oral glutamine in a 2005 Memorial Sloan Kettering study. The group receiving the l-glutamine had less weakness, less loss of vibratory sensation and less toe numbness.[111] The dose for helping to prevent neuropathy is 10 grams of l-glutamine powder taken 3 times per day for 5 days following IV chemotherapy. If you have chemotherapy on Sunday, then start the l-glutamine on Monday. You can mix l-glutamine in orange juice, water, yogurt or a smoothie. The flavor is quite bland and it dissolves well in liquids.

Phase	Chemotherapy		Side Effect	Neuropathy
Evidence Code	A		Dose	Preventative - 10 grams of powder taken 3 x daily for 5 days following IV chemotherapy

Do not take l-glutamine if your liver enzymes are more than double the normal upper limit, as this amino acid needs to be metabolised by the liver.

Alpha lipoic acid is a potent antioxidant and essential co-factor for metabolism of macronutrients to create energy. Your body can synthesise lipoic acid but the therapeutic level to treat neuropathy can only be achieved through supplementation. Also called thioctic acid, alpha lipoic acid significantly improved neuropathy at 600mg per day in a number of studies, as summarised in a recently published review article.[112] Some practitioners go as high as 600mg twice daily to treat chemotherapy-induced neuropathy.

Phase	Chemotherapy		Side Effect	Neuropathy
Evidence Code	A		Dose	600mg daily

Alpha lipoic acid can decrease blood sugar levels and should be used cautiously with uncontrolled diabetics and people with hypoglycemia so as not to cause hypoglycemia (low blood sugar).

Acetyl-l-carnitine is a form of l-carnitine that is more fat-soluble and therefore better at treating nerve and brain conditions. It has been shown to both prevent nerve damage and reverse existing numbness, pain and tingling as well as sensation loss. A 2007 review article suggested the cumulative evidence for acetyl-l-carnitine was sufficient to recommend use with paclitaxel and cisplatin.[113] The dose of acetyl-l-carnitine for prevention and treatment of neuropathy is 500mg taken twice daily.

Phase	Chemotherapy		Side Effect	Neuropathy
Evidence Code	A		Dose	Preventative 500mg twice daily

Note that Acetyl-L-Carnitine is not the same as L-Carnitine.

82

Hair and nail health

Chemotherapy and hormonal treatments can lead to hair loss (alopecia) and nail breakage and discolouration. Supporting the strength, health and re-growth of your hair and nails can help improve self-esteem and reduce self-consciousness during recovery.

Cooling gel cap & Gloves   Wearing a cooling gel cap during chemotherapy infusions can reduce drug seepage into the hair follicles and decrease hair loss. [114] [115] There are several systems for the cap, some involve using a portable refrigerator and others keep a steady temperature without refrigeration. The most common side effect from scalp cooling is headache. Wearing cool gloves or immersing your hands in ice water during chemotherapy can help prevent neuropathy and nail loss. The cold causes vasoconstriction of the vessels, preventing chemotherapy from saturating in your fingers. Patient with neuropathy of the feet can also wear cooling socks or submerge in ice water footbaths. One study also showed prevention of hand foot syndrome (palmar planter erythrodysthesia).[116]

Phase	Chemotherapy		Side Effect	Hair and nails
Evidence Code	A		Dose	Worn during every treatment

! *Scalp cooling is not appropriate for all cancers and should not be used if chemotherapy is given with a curative intent in patients with generalised haematogenic metastases.[117]*

Calcium, magnesium and zinc Calcium magnesium and zinc are minerals that contribute to nail and hair strength.[118]   A good supplement for hair and nails should have at least 15 mg of zinc, 200mg of magnesium and 400mg of calcium.

Phase	Chemotherapy		Side Effect	Hair and nails
Evidence Code	A		Dose	15mg zinc, 200mg magnesium and 400mg calcium daily

Essential Fatty Acids Essential fatty acids including Omega 3 and Omega 6 fats bring moisture and glossiness to hair and nails.[119]   Deficiency in these fats often manifest as hair, nail and skin problems.[120]   Dosing to prevent deficiency is 2000mg of combined EPA & DHA per day.

Phase	Chemotherapy		Side Effect	Hair and nails
Evidence Code	A		Dose	2000mg daily

Horsetail (Equisetum arvense) Horsetail (*Equisetum arvense*) is an herb rich in the nutrient silica, which is utilised by the body's hair, nails and teeth.[121]   Horsetail has been used historically for strengthening of connective tissue but also for kidney health as a diuretic. Equisetum has demonstrated anti-tumour activity in several animal studies.[122]   Dosing of the liquid extract is 30 drops twice daily of a 2:1 ration of plant to aqueous or alcohol extract. Dosing of the solid extract is 100mg twice daily.

Phase	Chemotherapy		Side Effect	Hair and nails
Evidence Code	BCD		Dose	100mg twice daily

Leukopenia & Neutropenia (Low WBC count)

Chemotherapy can cause suppression of the bone marrow, leading to a lower production of white blood cells, a low WBC count is known as Leukopenia & Neutropenia and leaves the body more vulnerable to infections, both from exposure in the community and to hospital acquired pathogens. There are drugs available to stimulate production of neutrophils, a type of white blood cell. The most common of these drugs is called Neulasta and it is often used concomitantly with chemotherapy. The most common side effect of Neulasta is deep bone pain, which can be quite intense and last from several hours up until a week or more.

Homeopathic Eupatorium. Homeopathic Eupatorium is prescribed by homeopaths and alternative practitioners to alleviate the bone pain from Neulasta. Homeopathy (www.homeopathic.org) is a 200 year old whole system of alternative medicine. Homeopathic remedies are chosen based on a variety of symptoms. These remedies are highly diluted and very safe. German research found homeopathic Eupatorium as effective as aspirin in controlling symptoms of the flu.[123] Take 3 pellets as often as needed to help with pain or soreness in your bones. The dose is 30 c, but you can increase to 200c if 30c is not strong enough or stops working as well as it did previously. Evidence Level D for drug-induced bone pain, Evidence Level A for flu aches and pains.

Phase	Chemotherapy	Side Effect	Low white blood cell count
Evidence Code	AD	Dose	30c dosage can be increased to 200c

AHCC (Active Hexose Correlated Compound) is a mixture of polysaccharides found in medicinal mushrooms that works to boost immune system function. It has been studied extensively for its anti-cancer properties, that works in part by stimulating the immune system but also has direct cancer inhibition properties. A Yale study of immune function in individuals over the age of 55 found AHCC increased CD4 helper cells, immune cells important for cytokine production. Japanese liver cancer patients given AHCC in a prospective study lived twice as long as those who did not receive the polysaccharides.[124] The AHCC group also had a lower recurrence rate. Dosing ranges vary for AHCC but generally for cancer or immune support, the dose is 1000mg (1 gram) taken twice daily. AHCC can be pricey but it's important to use a pure, high quality product.

Phase	Chemotherapy
Evidence Code	A

Side Effect	Low white blood cell count
Dose	1000mg twice daily

Thrombocytopenia (Low platelet count)

Platelets, which are produced by the bone marrow, is another type of blood cell that may be impacted by chemotherapy drugs.

Sesame oil has been used anecdotally to help with bone marrow production of platelets. This discovery was made when research veterinarians searched a food to boost low platelets in lab monkeys; sesame seeds and particularly the oil, was found to have the most benefit. Its use in humans for this purpose is not documented but as sesame is a food, its safety is excellent and the only known contraindication would be sesame allergy or a medically restricted low fat diet.

The dose is 1 teaspoon taken orally (by mouth) three times daily. An additional tablespoon should be applied topically to the thin parts of the skin as sesame oil can be absorbed transdermally. Sesame oil tastes good in stir fry, in tahini or humus or on salads mixed with vinegar for a dressing.

Phase	Chemotherapy		Side Effect	Low platelet count
Evidence Code	D		Dose	1 teaspoon x 3 times daily orally & 1 teaspoon topically

Homeopathic Phosphorus has been used to treat anaemias of all sorts including thrombocytopenia by classical homeopaths. It's supportive of the blood and should be taken at the 30c potency three times daily for this purpose. There has been no clinical trial to date showing benefit of using homeopathic to treat thrombocytopenia. Homeopathic medicines are very safe and have no known drug interactions.

Phase	Chemotherapy		Side Effect	Low platelet count
Evidence Code	D		Dose	30c potency 3 x daily

Papaya Leaf juice is used in South-east Asia and India to treat conditions of thrombocytopenia, primarily those caused by infections such as dengue fever, but it has also been used with cancer patients. There has been no definitive scholarly publication of human consumption of papaya leaf to explain the mechanism of action. A 2009 paper found increases of thrombocytes (platelets) in mice following consumption of papaya leaf in a palm oil suspension.[125] Traditionally papaya leaf juice is dosed frequently, approximately 20ml of the juice every two hours until thrombocytopenia resolves.

Phase	Chemotherapy		Side Effect	Low platelet count
Evidence Code	B		Dose	20mls every 2 hours

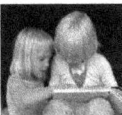

RADIATION - General

General radiation recommendations

Astragalus is an herb used in traditional Chinese medicine to support the immune system and prevent colds and flues. It has research to illustrate direct anti-tumour effects but is also indicated for use with radiation therapy. A recent study showed decreased organ damage and increased survival in mice treated with radiation.[126]
Dose: 3-6 grams per day in divided doses.
Typically, 2 grams three times daily.

Phase	Radiation -General
Evidence Code	B

Side Effect	Organ damage
Dose	3-6 grams/day eg. 2grams 3 x daily

Bioflavonoids (Quercetin/Genistein/Soy Isoflavone). The benefit of bioflavonoids for blood vessel healing after surgery was discussed in the previous section, but bioflavonoids also have been shown to decrease the side effects of radiation and can actually help make radiation more effective.

In a study involving flavonoid use with hepatoma (liver cancer) radiation, the flavonoids both increased the cancer cell death by reducing their ability to repair the radiation damage and they were directly anti-tumour.[127] The flavonoids in this study were genistein from soy, apigenin, and quercetin.

89

A radiation study involving patients with non-small cell lung cancer showed soy isoflavones to selectively inhibit the ability of cancer cells to repair.[128]

Quercetin dosing: 250mg daily -can be divided doses
Genistein/soy isoflavone dosing: 100mg twice daily

Quercetin and Genistein/soy isoflavone may be used independently or in combination. Genistein has synergy with the chemotherapy drug gemcitabine so is used for pancreatic and prostrate cancers. Quercetin has anti-cancer properties and is currently used for hematological malignancies. Any bioflavonoid is beneficial with radiation, however Quercetin and Genistein/Soy isoflavone are the most studied and most often used.

Phase	Radiation -General
Evidence Code	A

Side Effect	Cell damage/enhance radiation effect
Dose	**Quercetin**: 250mg daily **Genistein/soy isoflavone** 100mg twice daily

Curcumin extract comes from turmeric, a root used in Indian cooking that gives curry its characteristic yellow orange colour. This powerful herb has been shown to increase effectiveness and decrease inflammation. It is also strongly anti-tumour independent of its beneficial role for radiation.

A recent study found curcumin to significantly increase the death of neuroblastoma cancer cells (a type of brain tumor) exposed to ionising radiation.[129]

Phase	Radiation -General
Evidence Code	A

Side Effect	Inflammation/ enhance radiation effect
Dose	1500mg twice daily during treatment

Essential Fatty Acids-Omega 3: Much has been written in the popular press about the role of Omega 3 fatty acids in heart health, but they are also essential for decreasing inflammation and have well established anti-cancer benefit. During radiation, they decrease the incidence of side effects by reducing inflammation, swelling and irritation of healthy cells. They also have evidence for selectively increasing the cell death of cancer cells exposed to radiation therapy.

A 2011 German study demonstrated that EPA (Eicosapentaenoic Acid, a form of Omega 3 fatty acids), acted to radio sensitise both colon and glioblastoma (aggressive brain cancer) cells.[130] This means that the same amount of radiation killed cancer cells more effectively in the presence of Omega 3 fatty acids. Healthy cells did not have increased damage or death. The most common forms of Omega 3 fats are flaxseed, flaxseed oil, fish, and krill oils - all of which should be kept refrigerated.

Phase	Radiation -General
Evidence Code	A

Side Effect	Inflammation/ enhance radiation effect
Dose	1500mg twice daily during treatment

Check with your doctor before starting Omega 3 fats if you are on anti-coagulant therapy (blood thinners).

Ginkgo biloba extract is an herb that has been shown to reduce the damage to healthy cells without affecting the desired outcome in patients given radioactive iodine to treat Grave's disease.[131] Antioxidants in ginkgo biloba extract decreased the blood markers of radiation exposure in people occupationally exposed to ionising radiation.[132] Take 60mg twice daily, start 3-4 days before radiation and continue for 1 month after the completion of radiation.

Phase	Radiation -General		Side Effect	DNA damage
Evidence Code	A		Dose	60mg twice daily, start 3-4 days before & continue 1 month post treatment

Niacin in the form of niacinamide or nicotinamide has been shown to act as a radiosensitiser in radioiodine therapy for hyperthyroidism and thyroid cancer.[133] As a radiosensitiser, niacin increased blood flow and oxygen to the thyroid, which made cancer cell more susceptible to destruction from radiation. Oxygen is key to the destructive ability of radiation therapy and no increase in toxicity to healthy cells was observed as no additional side effects were reported in the groups given the niacinamide. The dose is 3-6 grams per day.

Phase	Radiation -General		Side Effect	Enhance radiation effectiveness
Evidence Code	A		Dose	3-6 grams daily

RADIATION – Specific sites

Breast radiation & any skin irritation

The most common side effect from whole breast radiation is a skin reaction. Patients can experience skin reddening and tenderness. If the irritation progresses, it can cause a breakdown of the skin with erosion of the top layer or layers of cells. Fortunately, there are some natural topical applications that can help decrease the incidence and severity of radiation dermatitis – the medical term for radiation skin reaction.

Calendula lotion helps to soothe dry, burned or irritated skin. Use it topically after radiation but not for four hours before. The reason to avoid using beforehand is that changes in the topography of the skin surface could theoretically alter the direction of the radiation beam. Apply 2-3 times per day after radiation treatment. A 2011 review article looking at radiation skin reactions showed calendula creams reduced the incidence of Grade 2 and 3 skin reactions. Grade 1 is the least severe and Grade 4 is the most severe.[134]

Phase	Radiation – Breast & Skin	Side Effect	Skin reactions
Evidence Code	A	Dose	Apply 2-3 times daily after radiation

Coconut oil is nourishing and very emollient. It is much thicker than the calendula lotions so it is best to apply after calendula lotion if both are being used at the same time. The same rules apply with the coconut oil: apply after radiation but not for four hours before. Studies have shown coconut oil to be as effective as mineral oil for moistening dry skin.[135] Apply 1-2 times per day to the affected area.

Phase	Radiation – Breast & Skin		Side Effect	Skin reactions
Evidence Code	A		Dose	Apply 1-2 times daily

Head/neck esophagus radiation

Honey (pure, natural) provides an anti-microbial role in head and neck cancers, but it also helps prevent radiation-induced mucositis. Manuka honey is the most well-studied type of honey but many studies have been done with plain, commercial honey. A Nepalese study showed honey to be superior to conventionally recommended lignocaine for the prevention of radiation-induced mucositis (mouth sores). The honey group had less incidence of mucositis and also less severity.[136] The minimum dosage for honey is 1 teaspoon taken 3 times daily. Do not take honey if you are unable to eat by mouth.

Phase	Radiation- Head/Neck Esophagus		Side Effect	Radiation induced mucositis
Evidence Code	A		Dose	1- teaspoon 3 times daily

L-glutamine powder can be used to help with healing of healthy gastrointestinal cells during and after radiation therapy.[137] Glutamine is necessary for repair of digestive tract tissues. Take 10 grams daily during radiation therapy. Ideally, the glutamine should be able to come in contact with the irritated area so powders and liquids are preferred to capsules for this purpose.

Phase	Radiation- Head/Neck Esophagus	Side Effect	Irritated digestive tract
Evidence Code	A	Dose	10 grams daily during treatment

Prostate radiation

Most prostate radiation is now well localised and there is now less damage to healthy tissues as the result of technological advances. However, depending on the location of the tumour(s) collateral damage can provoke urinary symptoms and radiation-induced proctitis, which is inflammation and irritation of the rectum. Natural medicines can help prevent some of these symptoms from occurring or reduce their severity. Please see the section on general radiation recommendations as well as the following.

Saw palmetto (Serenoa repens) is most commonly used to treat benign prostatic hyperplasia (BPH). The berries of saw palmetto inhibit 5-alpha reductase, an enzyme which produces dihydrotestosterone (DHT). DHT and 5-alpha reductase are higher in prostate tissue with BPH and contribute to urinary disturbances. In studies, saw palmetto inhibited the enzyme responsible for making DHT – in that way, it also decreased the levels of DHT, reducing urinary symptoms in men, including frequency, urgency and flow.[138] Saw palmetto is also a strong anti-inflammatory, reducing swelling and pain in irritated tissues.[139]

Phase	Radiation- Prostate		Side Effect	Urinary symptoms
Evidence Code	A		Dose	160mg twice daily

Slippery Elm Bark can be used to soothe the urinary tract. Slippery elm is demulcent, which means that it helps coat a healing film over irritated mucus membranes. Mix 1 teaspoon of the powder into a water, tea or juice and drink 2-3 times daily. Slippery elm is also utilised in the treatment of irritable bowel syndrome. An Australian study found it helpful, in combination with other herbs, for improving symptoms of irritable bowel syndrome, particularly those with constipation predominant IBS.[140]

Phase	Radiation- Prostate		Side Effect	Urinary tract irritation
Evidence Code	AD		Dose	1 teaspoon 2-3 times daily

Radiation to bones

Homeopathic Eupatorium is indicated to help with bone pain. It is safe, gentle and does not interact with other medications. Starting dose is 3 pellets of 30c potency taken as needed to help with bone pain. There is no clinical study to date showing Homeopathic Eupatorium to be effective in reducing cancer-associated bone pain. This recommendation is based on historical use.

Phase	Radiation- Bones		Side Effect	Bone pain
Evidence Code	D		Dose	3 pellets 30c taken as needed

Nutritional support can help support bone strength & reduce the risk of fracture. Vitamin D, calcium, magnesium, & essential fatty acids (fish/krill oils) all play important roles in bone health.

Vitamin D The dose of Vitamin D for bone health is 1000 IU per day. Men with higher blood level of Vitamin D at prostate cancer diagnosis had better outcomes than those with lower Vitamin D status.[141]

Phase	Radiation- Bones		Side Effect	Weak bone/risk of fracture
Evidence Code	A		Dose	1000IU daily

Calcium The dose of calcium is 800mg per day if a person is eating some calcium rich foods, if not then the dose should be 1200mg per day.

Phase	Radiation- Bones		Side Effect	Weak bone/risk of fracture
Evidence Code	A		Dose	800-1200mg daily

Magnesium should be dosed between 300 and 500mg per day to support bone health, depending on dietary intake of magnesium foods and magnesium loss.

Note: Patients recovering from orthopedic limb surgery reported less pain and required less morphine use when given supplemental intravenous magnesium sulfate.[142]

Phase	Radiation- Bones		Side Effect	Weak bone/risk of fracture
Evidence Code	A		Dose	300-500mg daily

Essential Fatty Acids - Omega 3 Cancer patients undergoing radiation need 1500mg of EPA Omega 3 fatty acids twice daily. Check with your doctor before starting Omega 3 fats if you are on anti-coagulant therapy (blood thinners).

Phase	Radiation- Bones		Side Effect	Weak bone/risk of fracture
Evidence Code	A		Dose	1500mg twice daily

⚠️ *Check with your GP before starting Omega 3 fats if you 're on anti-coagulant therapy (blood thinners).*

Abdominal or pelvic radiation

Vitamin A helps the healing of epithelial cells. It is essential for wound healing and immune function.[143] Radiation to the abdomen, depending on the path of the beam arcs, can cause irritation to the rectum. This condition is called radiation proctitis. Used short term during radiation and the following weeks, dosing is 25,000 IU taken twice daily.

Phase	Radiation- Abdominal/ Pelvic		Side Effect	Proctitis
Evidence Code	A		Dose	25000IU twice daily during & couple wks post treatment

Do not take high doses of Vitamin A long term without doctor supervision as it is a fat soluble vitamin and can bioaccumulate.

Berberine is an herb commonly used to treat infections and has some new research showing benefit in diabetes mellitus. In patients undergoing abdominal radiation, berberine was shown in a human study to reduce damage to intestines.[144] The dosing for radiation is 200mg twice daily.

Phase	Radiation- Abdominal/ Pelvic		Side Effect	Damage to intestines
Evidence Code	A		Dose	200mg twice daily

Brain radiation

Boswelia is an herb used traditionally to treat inflammatory, rheumatic conditions. A recent, very strong study showed boswelia reduced swelling in the brain in patients who received brain radiation; 60 per cent of patients taking boswelia had a 75 per cent or greater reduction in swelling as compared to only 26 per cent in the placebo group.[145] In the study 4200mg of boswelia was given per day. This would be roughly 2 grams twice daily.

Phase	Radiation- Brain		Side Effect	Brain swelling
Evidence Code	A		Dose	4200mg daily / 2 grams twice daily

Bacopa is an herb that enhances memory and cognition. Forgetfulness and brain fog are two of the most common complaints of patients undergoing brain radiation or who recently completed radiation therapy. A randomised, double bind, placebo-controlled study of older Australians found Bacopa significantly improved new memory acquisition, verbal learning, and delayed recall of facts.[146] Extracts of bacopa have also been studied to improve symptoms of fatigue by increasing stamina. The dose for improving mental function is 200mg twice daily.

Phase	Radiation- Brain		Side Effect	Brain fog/ memory loss
Evidence Code	A		Dose	200mg twice daily

Hematological malignancies

Leukemia, lymphoma, and multiple myeloma are cancers of the blood and lymph nodes. Since these cells comprise part of your immune system, there is debate among the integrative oncology community about the role of immune supportive therapies. Some worry that an herb or nutrient that stimulates the immune system could stimulate the growth of even more cancer cells.

Others point to research showing that natural therapies can selectively stimulate only the growth of healthy cells and not cancerous cells. A 2005 study of Chinese children with acute leukemia were given large doses of astragalus root, 90 grams daily for one month. Those children receiving the astragalus had nearly twice the number of dendritic cells, which are immune cells that help your body identify hazardous cells (antigens), which in the case of leukemia are the cancerous cells.[147]

An animal study showed the immune stimulating herb Echinacea extended survival in mice with leukemia.[148] In Europe, there is widespread use of the immune stimulating herb mistletoe, also called Viscum Album, and formulated for injection under the names Helixor and Iscador. Ironically, some published case studies and pre-clinical data (cell line and animal studies) have shown benefit in some patient populations with leukemia and lymphomas. A Swiss cell study from 2008 showed mistletoe formula Iscador to be as effective as the standard chemotherapy Vincristine against human B cell lymphoma.[149]

It's premature to suggest that people with hematological malignancies are completely safe to take immune stimulating herbs and nutrients. Ongoing research will hopefully give greater understanding of the role of immune stimulation versus immune modulation, the later being a selective influence on immune function and not fueling growth of cancer cells.

Immune stimulating herbs, nutrients & mushrooms

The following are applicable for all treatment phases, however ensure you investigate any possible drug interactions with your treatment medication as explained in the next section.

Echinacea[150]

Dose	300mg three x daily	Evidence Code	A

Astragalus[151]

Dose	1.5 grams twice daily	Evidence Code	A

Maitake [152]

Dose	50mg three x daily	Evidence Code	A

Shitake [153]

Dose	4 grams daily	Evidence Code	A

Reishi[154]

Dose	1.5 grams three times daily		Evidence Code	A

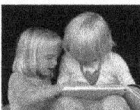

Mistletoe[155]

Dose	1ml injected 2-3 times per week		Evidence Code	A

St. John's wort[156]

Dose	300mg three x daily		Evidence Code	A

AHCC[157]

Dose	1 gram three x daily		Evidence Code	A

Beta glucan[158]

Dose	250mg 1-2 times daily		Evidence Code	A

Cat's Claw[159]

Dose	350mg daily		Evidence Code	A

CHEMOTHERAPY INTERACTIONS WITH NATURAL AGENTS

As mentioned at the <u>beginning of this section</u>, it is important to understand that some natural substances can interact with certain drugs and medication to make them more active or inactive. As the primary sites of transformation are the liver and intestines, we have provided the following tables to highlight those natural agents and cancer drugs that have an interaction either inducing or inhibiting. These tables are probably best shared with your oncologist and other health care professionals.

Here is an example of how to use the table on the next page to identify the natural agents that can interact with your drug.

If you were using Tamoxifen, the table lists American Ginseng, Asian Ginseng, Siberian Ginseng, St. John's Wort, Gingko as natural substances that may induce the CYP enzymes speeding up drug metabolism and potentially decreasing the concentration or effectiveness of the drug.

On the other hand, the table list the natural agents Devil's Claw, Garlic, Ginkgo, Gotu Kola, Quercetin, Resveratrol, Soy, Isoflavones, Reishi, Garlic, Kava Kava as substances that may inhibit the CYP enzymes, slowing down drug metabolism and potentially increasing levels of chemotherapeutic drug.

If you are taking...Tamoxifen

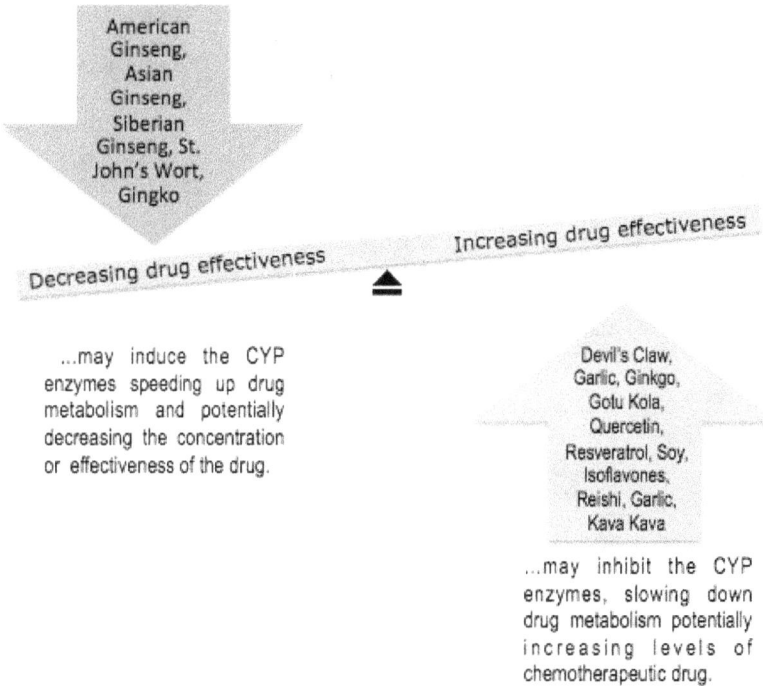

American Ginseng, Asian Ginseng, Siberian Ginseng, St. John's Wort, Gingko

Decreasing drug effectiveness

Increasing drug effectiveness

...may induce the CYP enzymes speeding up drug metabolism and potentially decreasing the concentration or effectiveness of the drug.

Devil's Claw, Garlic, Ginkgo, Gotu Kola, Quercetin, Resveratrol, Soy, Isoflavones, Reishi, Garlic, Kava Kava

...may inhibit the CYP enzymes, slowing down drug metabolism potentially increasing levels of chemotherapeutic drug.

ACTION

Make a list of the drugs you are currently on, then review the following table for natural agents that may induce or inhibit CYP enzymes either reducing or increasing drug effectiveness. Keep this list close by to refer to as you investigate the natural agents listed in this book to help in managing your side effects.

Note: you will have to review this list as your medication changes.

Interactions of Chemotherapeutic Agents and Natural Products with Liver Enzyme

CYP (Liver Enzymes) ↓	Chemotherapy, Hormone therapy or Targeted therapy ↓	Natural Inducers (Speed up drug metabolism, potentially decreasing levels of chemotherapeutic drug) ↓	Natural Inhibitors (Slow down drug metabolism, potentially increasing levels of chemotherapeutic drug) ↓
No known CYP substrate	Bevacizumab Carboplatin Cetuximab Gemcitabine Methotrexate Temozolomide Trastuzumab Sunitinib		
1A2	Dacarbazine Etoposide Fluorouracil Ifosfamide Imatinib Bortezomib Oxaliplatin Toremifene	Resveratrol St. John's Wort Sulphorophanes Broccoli sprouts	Ginkgo Echinacea Reishi
2A6	Fluorouracil Ifosfamide Letrozole Tamoxifen Thalidomide		
2B6	Ifosfamide Irinotecan Tamoxifen Thalidomide		
2C8	Fluorouracil Ifosfamide Paclitaxel Thalidomide		Quercetin
2C9	Ifosfamide Paclitaxel Tamoxifen Thalidomide	American Ginseng Asian Ginseng Siberian Ginseng St. John's Wort	Devil's Claw Garlic Ginkgo Gotu Kola Quercetin Resveratrol Soy Isoflavones

106

Interactions of Chemotherapeutic Agents and Natural Products with Liver Enzyme			
CYP (Liver Enzymes) ↓	Chemotherapy, Hormone therapy or Targeted therapy ↓	Natural Inducers (Speed up drug metabolism, potentially decreasing levels of chemotherapeutic drug) ↓	Natural Inhibitors (Slow down drug metabolism, potentially increasing levels of chemotherapeutic drug) ↓
3A4	Docetaxel Doxorubicin Etoposide Everolimus Fulvestrant Ifosfamide Irinotecan Letrozole Paclitaxel Sorafenib Topotecan Tamoxifen Toremifene Vinblastine	American Ginseng Asian Ginseng Siberian Ginseng St. John's Wort	American Ginseng Cat's Claw Garlic Ginkgo Goldenseal Gotu Kola Grape Seed Grapefruit Green Tea Milk Thistle Mistletoe Quercetin Reishi Resveratrol Rhodiola Saw Palmetto Siberian Ginseng Valerian
3A5	Docetaxel Doxorubicin Etoposide Ifosfamide Irinotecan Paclitaxel Tamoxifen Vinblastine		

CYP Data sourced from PharmacologyWeekly.com, NaturalDatabase.com, the Super CYP database and Memorial Sloan-Kettering Herbal Monographs. The level of evidence of some of this CYP data is in vitro data, meaning observed influence in the lab petri dish and not in animals or humans. What can be extrapolated from this pre-clinical data is uncertain. It is important to consider any influence on drug metabolism when making decisions about using botanical medicine. That said, *nearly every food or beverage could also potentially affect chemotherapy metabolism.* A classic example of dietary interaction is the chemotherapy imatinib (Gleevec), which is metabolised down the same enzymatic pathway as caffeine. Patients can drink coffee, tea or caffeinated sodas during their imatinib infusions and this intake is not routinely restricted. Yet, those same patients are forbidden from taking any herbal supplements - even a few days later when the chemotherapy has already been fully metabolised.

To be cautious, one can look up or ask their practitioner for the half-life of their chemotherapy to determine how long the drug will be active in their body and then wait at least two full half lives before and after chemotherapy to use herbal medicine metabolised down the same CYP 450 enzymatic pathway. A "half-life" is the time it takes for half of the drug to eliminated by the body.

Websites with half-life information about drugs include RxList – The Internet Drug Index (www.rxlist.com) and Drugs.com – Drug Information Online (www.drugs.com) as well as the manufacturer of your medications. A naturopathic physician or integrative medical doctor trained in oncology can help you make safe, effective decisions for botanical use during active treatment.

Some drugs are not metabolised by CYP 450 enzymes, including chemotherapy. If you don't see your treatment medications listed in the table above, then check with your doctor or a reputable website such as those listed above.

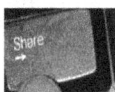

Wanting to share this book?
Email www.managesideeffectsofchemo.com to family & friends.

SECTION V: APPENDICES

Appendix 1: Table of natural supplements by treatment phase/side effect

EVIDENCE CODE & CAUTION KEY

A- Clinical Evidence in Humans

B- Animal Studies

C- In vitro evidence from observation made of cancer cells in a petri dish in a lab

D-Historical or traditional use

CA – identifies if there is a caution related to the natural supplement, please refer to the appropriate section of the book for further details

Surgery

TREATMENT PHASE	SIDE EFFECT	NATURAL SUPPLEMENT	DOSE	EVIDENCE CODE
Surgery	Healing	Zinc	15mg/day for 1 month post surgery	A
		Vitamin C	1000mg x 3 times daily for 1 month post surgery	A
		Bioflavonoids	200mg twice daily	A
		Bromelain	500mg 2-3times daily for 3-4 wks post surgery	A
	Reducing the spread of cancer cells -metastasis	Modified Citrus Pectin (MCP)	5mg x 3times daily for 1 wk prior & 1 mnth post surgery/biopsy	AB
	Reducing pain, swelling and bruising	Homeopathic Arnica	2-3 pellets under tongue 3-4 times daily or as needed post surgery	A
	Emotional support	Homeopathic Phosphorus	2-3 pellets of 30c potency under tongue as needed prior to surgery	D
		Homeopathic Gelsemium	2-3 pellets of 30c potency under tongue as needed prior to surgery	D
		Rescue Remedy	Liquid, pellets or spray – follow directions on label	D

Chemotherapy & hormone therapy

TREATMENT PHASE	SIDE EFFECT	NATURAL SUPPLEMENT	DOSE	EVIDENCE CODE	
Chemo & Hormone Therapies	Cardiotoxicity, fatigue	CoQ10	100mg twice daily	A	
		L-Carnitine	500mg twice daily	A	
		Taurine	1000-2000mg daily in divided doses	B	
	Constipation	Hydration (water)	Gen health- drink 1/2 body weight in ounces /day. A 200-pound person should drink 100 ounces /day.	A	
		Magnesium Citrate	150-300mg daily, higher doses	A	CA
		Probiotics	At least 5 billion cells daily	A	CA
	Diarrhea	L-Glutamine	10grams daily	A	
		Probiotics	At least 5 billion cells	A	
		Charcoal capsules	Starting dose is 600mg 3 x daily, increase up to 2400mg 3 x daily	A	
	Fatigue	L-Carnitine	1000mg x 3 times daily with meals	A	
		B Vitamins	1 capsule B complex daily or twice daily with meals	A	
		CoQ10	100-200mg daily	A	
	Fatigue (Stress)	Rhodiola rosea	100-200mg morning & afternoon (start with 100mg)	A	
		Astragalus	2grams x 3 daily	A	
	Hand Foot Syndrome (PPE)	Vitamin B6	300mg daily (or 3 x 100mg)	A	
		Antiperspirant deodorant	Apply twice daily	A	
		Aggressive skin hydration	Use liberally or thick cream at night	AD	
		Henna	Use 4 x daily	A	
		Topical DMSO	Use 4 x daily	A	
	Hot Flushes	Black Cohosh	80-100mg twice daily	A	
		Vitamin C	1000mg 3 x daily	A	
		Hesperidin	250mg 3 x daily	A	
		5-HTP	50-100mg 3 x daily	D	CA
		Soy Isoflavones	12-20grams of soy protein or 50mg of soy isoflavones daily	A	
		Magnesium	400 to 800mg daily in divided doses	A	

TREATMENT PHASE	SIDE EFFECT	NATURAL SUPPLEMENT	DOSE	EVIDENCE CODE	
Chemo & Hormone Therapies	Insomnia	*Melatonin*	1. Sleep-3-5mg 30 min before desired bed time 2. Anti Cancer- 20mg 30 min before desired bed time	A	
		Theanine	100mg 30 with dinner or before bed	A	
		Inositol	3-6grams daily & increase up to 6 grams. For sleep take 1 gram 1 hr prior to bed	A	
	Joint pain	*Bromelain*	200mg twice daily	A	
		Glucosamine & Chondroitin	1500mg glucosamine and 1000mg chondroitin daily	A	
		MSM	1000mg x 3 times daily	A	
		Curcumin	1000mg x 3-4 times daily	A	
	Mouth sores	*Honey*	1 tea -1 tablespoon applied to sore areas 3-4 times daily. Can also be added to food and eaten.	A	
		L-Glutamine	10 grams in 4 ounces of water & rinse mouth OR make a paste and apply	A	
		DGL	Apply to mouth sores	AD	
	Neuropathy	*Vitamin B6*	300mg daily with food	A	
		L-Glutamine	Preventative - 10 grams of powder taken 3 x daily for 5 days following IV chemotherapy	A	*CA*
		Alpha Lipoic Acid	600mg daily	A	*CA*
		Acetyl-L-Carnitine	Preventative 500mg twice daily	A	
	Low white blood cell count	*Homeopathic Eupatorium*	30c dosage can be increased to 200c	AD	
		AHCC	1000mg twice daily	A	
	Low platelet count	*Sesame oil*	1 teaspoon x 3 times daily orally & 1 teaspoon topically	D	
		Homeopathic Phosphorus	30c potency 3 x daily	D	
		Papaya Leaf	20mls every 2 hours	B	

TREATMENT PHASE	SIDE EFFECT	NATURAL SUPPLEMENT	DOSE	EVIDENCE CODE	
Chemo & Hormone Therapies	Hair and nail health	Cooling gel cap	Worn during every treatment	A	CA
		Calcium, Magnesium & Zinc	15mg zinc, 200mg magnesium and 400mg calcium daily	A	
		Essential Fatty Acids (Omega3,6)	2000mg daily	A	
		Horsetail	100mg twice daily	BCD	

Radiation – general & specific sites

TREATMENT PHASE	SIDE EFFECT	NATURAL SUPPLEMENT	DOSE	EVIDENCE CODE	
Radiation	Organ damage	Astragalus	3-6 grams/day eg. 2grams 3 x daily	B	
	Cell damage/enhance radiation effect	Genistein/Soy Isoflavone	Genistein/soy isoflavone 100mg twice daily	A	
		Quercetin	250mg daily	A	
	Inflammation/ enhance radiation effect	Curcumin	1500mg twice daily during treatment	A	
		Essential Fatty Acids- Omega 3 fats	1500mg twice daily during treatment	A	CA
	DNA damage	Ginkgo biloba extract	60mg twice daily, start 3-4 days before & continue 1 month post treatment	A	
	Enhance radiation effectiveness	Niacin	3-6 grams daily	A	

TREATMENT PHASE	SIDE EFFECT	NATURAL SUPPLEMENT	DOSE	EVIDENCE CODE
Radiation-Breast & Skin	Skin reactions	*Calendula lotion*	Apply 2-3 times daily	A
		Coconut Oil	Apply 1-2 times daily	A
Radiation-Head/Neck Esophagus	Radiation induced mucositis	*Honey*	1- teaspoon 3 times daily	A
	Irritated digestive tract	*L-Glutamine*	10 grams daily during treatment	A
Radiation-Prostate	Urinary symptoms	*Saw Palmetto*	160mg twice daily	A
	Urinary tract irritation	*Slippery Elm Bark*	1 teaspoon 2-3 times daily	AD
Radiation-Bones	Bone pain	*Homeopathic Eupatorium*	3 pellets 30c taken as needed	D
	Weak bone/risk of fracture	*Vitamin D*	1000IU daily	A
		Calcium	800-1200mg daily	A
		Magnesium	300-500mg daily	A
		Essential Fatty Acids- Omega 3	1500mg twice daily	A
Radiation-Abdominal / Pelvic	Proctitis	*Vitamin A*	25000IU twice daily during & couple wks post treatment	A
	Damage to intestines	*Berberine*	200mg twice daily	A
Radiation-Brain	Brain swelling	*Boswelia*	4200mg daily / 2 grams twice daily	A
	Brain fog/ memory loss	*Bacopa*	200mg twice daily	A

CA

CA

113

All treatment phases

TREATMENT PHASE	SIDE EFFECT	NATURAL SUPPLEMENT	DOSE	EVIDENCE CODE
All	Weak immune system	Echinacea	300mg three x daily	A
		Astragalus	1.5 grams twice daily	A
		Maitake	50mg three x daily	A
		Shitake	4 grams daily	A
		Reishi	1.5 grams three times daily	A
		Mistletoe	1ml injected 2-3 times per week	A
		St. John's Wort	300mg three x daily	A
		AHCC	1 gram three x daily	A
		Beta Glucan	250mg 1-2 times daily	A
		Cat's Claw	350mg daily	A

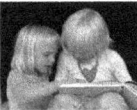

Appendix 2. Table of natural supplements A-Z

NATURAL SUPPLEMENT	TREATMENT PHASE	SIDE EFFECT	DOSE	EVIDENCE CODE	
5-HTP	Chemo	Hot Flushes	50-100mg 3 x daily	D	CA
Acetyl-L-Carnitine	Chemo	Neuropathy	Preventative 500mg twice daily	A	
Aggressive skin hydration	Chemo	Hand Foot Syndrome (PPE)	Use liberally or thick cream at night	AD	
AHCC	All	Weak immune system	1 gram three x daily	A	
AHCC	Chemo	Low white blood cell count	1000mg twice daily	A	
Alpha Lipoic Acid	Chemo	Neuropathy	600mg daily	A	CA
Antiperspirant deodorant	Chemo	Hand Foot Syndrome (PPE)	Apply twice daily	A	
Astragalus	Chemo	Fatigue (Stress)	2grams x 3 daily	A	
Astragalus	All	Weak immune system	1.5 grams twice daily	A	
Astragalus	Radiation	Organ damage	3-6 grams/day eg. 2grams 3 x daily	B	
B Vitamins	Chemo	Fatigue	1 capsule B complex daily or twice daily with meals	A	
Bacopa	Radiation- Brain	Brain fog/ memory loss	200mg twice daily	A	
Berberine	Radiation- Abdominal/ Pelvic	Damage to intestines	200mg twice daily	A	
Beta Glucan	All	Weak immune system	250mg 1-2 times daily	A	
Bioflavonoids	Surgery	Healing	200mg twice daily	A	
Black Cohosh	Chemo	Hot Flushes	80-100mg twice daily	A	
Boswelia	Radiation- Brain	Brain swelling	4200mg daily / 2 grams twice daily	A	
Bromelain	Surgery	Healing	500mg 2-3times daily for 3-4 wks post surgery	A	
Bromelain	Chemo	Joint pain	200mg twice daily	A	

115

NATURAL SUPPLEMENT	TREATMENT PHASE	SIDE EFFECT	DOSE	EVIDENCE CODE	
Calcium	Radiation- Bones	Weak bone/risk of fracture	800-1200mg daily	A	
Calcium, Magnesium & Zinc	Chemo & Hormone Therapies	Hair and nail health	15mg zinc, 200mg magnesium and 400mg calcium daily	A	
Calendula lotion	Radiation- Breast & Skin	Skin reactions	Apply 2-3 times daily	A	
Cat's Claw	All	Weak immune system	350mg daily	A	
Charcoal capsules	Chemo	Diarrhea	Starting dose is 600mg 3 x daily, increase up to 2400mg 3 x daily	A	
Coconut Oil	Radiation- Breast & Skin	Skin reactions	Apply 1-2 times daily	A	
Cooling gel cap	Chemo & Hormone Therapies	Hair and nail health	Worn during every treatment	A	CA
CoQ10	Chemo	Cardiotoxicity, fatigue	100mg twice daily	A	
	Chemo	Fatigue	100-200mg daily	A	
Curcumin	Chemo	Joint pain	1000mg x 3-4 times daily	A	
	Radiation	Inflammation/ enhance radiation effect	1500mg twice daily during treatment	A	
DGL	Chemo	Mouth sores	Apply to mouth sores	AD	
Echinacea	All	Weak immune system	300mg three x daily	A	
Essential Fatty Acids (Omega3,6)	Chemo & Hormone Therapies	Hair and nail health	2000mg daily	A	
	Radiation- Bones	Weak bone/risk of fracture	1500mg twice daily	A	CA
	Radiation	Inflammation/ enhance radiation effect	1500mg twice daily during treatment	A	CA

116

NATURAL SUPPLEMENT	TREATMENT PHASE	SIDE EFFECT	DOSE	EVIDENCE CODE
Genistein/ Soy Isoflavone	Radiation	Cell damage/enhance radiation effect	Genistein/soy isoflavone 100mg twice daily	A
Ginkgo biloba extract	Radiation	DNA damage	60mg twice daily, start 3-4 days before & continue 1 month post treatment	A
Glucosamine & Chondroitin	Chemo	Joint pain	1500mg glucosamine and 1000mg chondroitin daily	A
Henna	Chemo	Hand Foot Syndrome (PPE)	Use 4 x daily	A
Hesperidin	Chemo	Hot Flushes	250mg 3 x daily	A
Homeopathic Arnica	Surgery	Reducing pain, swelling and bruising	2-3 pellets under tongue 3-4 times daily or as needed post surgery	A
Homeopathic Eupatorium	Chemo	Low white blood cell count	30c dosage can be increased to 200c	AD
	Radiation-Bones	Bone pain	3 pellets 30c taken as needed	D
Homeopathic Gelsemium	Surgery	Emotional support	2-3 pellets of 30c potency under tongue as needed prior to surgery	D
Homeopathic Phosphorus	Surgery	Emotional support	2-3 pellets of 30c potency under tongue as needed prior to surgery	D
	Chemo	Low platelet count	30c potency 3 x daily	D

NATURAL SUPPLEMENT	TREATMENT PHASE	SIDE EFFECT	DOSE	EVIDENCE CODE
Honey	Chemo	Mouth sores	1 tea -1 tablespoon applied to sore areas 3-4 times daily. Can also be added to food and eaten.	A
Honey	Radiation-Head/Neck Esophagus	Radiation induced mucositis	1- teaspoon 3 times daily	A
Horsetail	Chemo & Hormone Therapies	Hair and nail health	100mg twice daily	BCD
Hydration (water)	Chemo	Constipation	Gen health- drink 1/2 body weight in ounces /day. A 200-pound person should drink 100 ounces /day.	A
Inositol	Chemo	Insomnia	3-6grams daily & increase up to 6 grams. For sleep take 1 gram 1 hr prior to bed	A
L-Carnitine	Chemo	Cardiotoxicity, fatigue	500mg twice daily	A
	Chemo	Fatigue	1000mg x 3 times daily with meals	A

NATURAL SUPPLEMENT	TREATMENT PHASE	SIDE EFFECT	DOSE	EVIDENCE CODE	
L-Glutamine	Chemo	Diarrhea	10grams daily	A	
	Chemo	Mouth sores	10 grams in 4 ounces of water & rinse mouth OR make a paste and apply	A	
	Chemo	Neuropathy	Preventative – 10 grams of powder taken 3 x daily for 5 days following IV chemotherapy	A	CA
	Radiation-Head/Neck Esophagus	Irritated digestive tract	10 grams daily during treatment	A	
Magnesium	Chemo	Hot Flushes	400 to 800mg daily in divided doses	A	
	Radiation-Bones	Weak bone/risk of fracture	300-500mg daily	A	
Magnesium Citrate	Chemo	Constipation	150-300mg daily, higher doses	A	CA
Maitake	All	Weak immune system	50mg three x daily	A	
Melatonin	Chemo	Insomnia	1. Sleep-3-5mg 30 min before desired bed time 2. Anti Cancer-20mg 30 min before desired bed time	A	
Mistletoe	All	Weak immune system	1ml injected 2-3 times per week	A	

NATURAL SUPPLEMENT	TREATMENT PHASE	SIDE EFFECT	DOSE	EVIDENCE CODE
Modified Citrus Pectin (MCP)	Surgery	Reducing the spread of cancer cells - metastasis	5mg x 3times daily for 1 wk prior & 1 mnth post surgery/biopsy	AB
MSM	Chemo	Joint pain	1000mg x 3 times daily	A
Niacin	Radiation	Enhance radiation effectiveness	3-6 grams daily	A
Papaya Leaf	Chemo	Low platelet count	20mls every 2 hours	B
Probiotics	Chemo	Constipation	At least 5 billion cells daily	A
	Chemo	Diarrhea	At least 5 billion cells	A
Quercetin	Radiation	Cell damage/enhance radiation effect	250mg daily	A
Reishi	All	Weak immune system	1.5 grams three times daily	A
Rescue Remedy	Surgery	Emotional support	Liquid, pellets or spray – follow directions on label	D
Rhodiola rosea	Chemo	Fatigue (Stress)	100-200mg morning & afternoon (start with 100mg)	A
Saw Palmetto	Radiation-Prostate	Urinary symptoms	160mg twice daily	A
Sesame oil	Chemo	Low platelet count	1 teaspoon x 3 times daily orally & 1 teaspoon topically	D
Shitake	All	Weak immune system	4 grams daily	A
Slippery Elm Bark	Radiation-Prostate	Urinary tract irritation	1 teaspoon 2-3 times daily	AD

CA

NATURAL SUPPLEMENT	TREATMENT PHASE	SIDE EFFECT	DOSE	EVIDENCE CODE
Soy Isoflavones	Chemo	Hot Flushes	12-20grams of soy protein or 50mg of soy isoflavones daily	A
St. John's Wort	All	Weak immune system	300mg three x daily	A
Taurine	Chemo	Cardiotoxicity, fatigue	1000-2000mg daily in divided doses	B
Theanine	Chemo	Insomnia	100mg 30 with dinner or before bed	A
Topical DMSO	Chemo	Hand Foot Syndrome (PPE)	Use 4 x daily	A
Vitamin A	Radiation-Abdominal/Pelvic	Proctitis	25000IU twice daily during & couple wks post treatment	A
Vitamin B6	Chemo	Neuropathy	300mg daily with food	A
Vitamin B6	Chemo	Hand Foot Syndrome (PPE)	300mg daily (or 3 x 100mg)	A
Vitamin C	Surgery	Healing	1000mg x 3 times daily for 1 month post surgery	A
Vitamin C	Chemo	Hot Flushes	1000mg 3 x daily	A
Vitamin D	Radiation-Bones	Weak bone/risk of fracture	1000IU daily	A
Zinc	Surgery	Healing	15mg/day for 1 month post surgery	A

CA

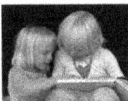

Appendix 3. Tips on finding integrative oncology providers

1. **Naturopathic physicians** specialising in oncology have the most advanced training in natural treatments for cancer care. Naturopathic doctors have ND or NMD after their name. They are designated with acronym FABNO that stands for Fellow of the American Board of Naturopathic Oncology. You can find a FABNO certified naturopathic physician at the OncANP website (www.oncanp.org). A listing of naturopathic physicians is available on the American Association of Naturopathic Physician's website. (www.naturopathic.org) Both websites have international listings.

2. **Holistic medical doctors** and osteopathic physicians with advanced training in natural or integrative medicine may specialise in cancer care. Look for information regarding practitioners with oncology qualifications on the following websites

   a. Canadian Association for Integrative & Energy Therapies (www.caiet.org)

   b. American Holistic Medical Association (www.holisticmedicine.org)

   c. American College for Advancement in Medicine, (www.acamnet.org)

   d. British Society of Integrated Medicine (www.bsim.org.uk)

   e. Australian Integrative Medicine Association (www.aima.net.au)

3. **Acupuncturists** can help with a variety of ailments including host flushes, fatigue and neuropathy. Insurance coverage for acupuncture has increased dramatically in the past decade, minimising out of pocket costs for the treatments. There are websites that can help you find a acupuncturist or Chinese herbalist for most countries, here are the links for
   a. Canada (www.acufinder.com/Acupuncture)
   b. USA (www.nccaom.org/find-an-acupuncture-practitioner-directory)
   c. UK (www.acupuncture-practitioners.co.uk)
   d. Australia. (www.acupuncture.org.au)
4. **Registered Dieticians** specialising in hospital nutrition or cancer nutrition can help patients make meal plans or adjust diet to side effects and treatments. For example, there are dietary modifications that can help with constipation, diarrhea or reflux. Your local hospital may have registered dieticians on staff or you can search for one online with the
   a. Eat Right Organisation for the USA (www.eatright.org)
   b. Dietitians of Canada (www.dietitians.ca),
   c. British Dietetic Association (www.bda.uk.com)
   d. Dietitians Association of Australia. (www.daa.asn.au /for-the-public/)

Appendix 4. Where to buy natural supplements

If you're like me, you can get mighty confused when searching for a supplement that is not run of the mill, for example Bacop. First you have to find out what it is: is it a herb or a mineral? A quick visit to Wikipedia sorts that out, then what form does it come in? What are the processing issues so you can ensure you get the best quality? Is it organic? What quantities will I need to buy?

Well, we can help you with a few of those questions as our wise naturopathic physicians have provided a sample of professional and reputable supplement companies that adhere to Current Good Manufacturing Practice Guidelines for us. And to be honest, when you're undergoing cancer treatment, you rarely have the energy, time or head space to find these products... so hopefully we have saved you some time and effort with the list of links below.

Interesting, you can only purchase online from a number of these reputable supplement companies if you are a practitioner or have a doctor's code, which is not always easy to organise. However, we have sourced a few online websites where you can purchase these reputable products directly, without being a practitioner.

A <u>sample</u> of professional supplement companies that adhere to current good manufacturing practice guidelines:

1. Bach flower essences
2. Boiron Homeopathics
3. Carlson Labs
4. Gaia Herbs
5. Helios Homeopathics
6. Herb Pharm
7. Innate Response
8. Integrative Therapeutics
9. Klaire Labs
10. Metabolic Maintenance
11. Metagenics
12. Nordic Naturals
13. Pharmax
14. Progressive Labs
15. Pure Encapsulations
16. Thorne
17. Vital Nutrients
18. Vitanica

The table below is a comprehensive list of all supplements and where you can purchase them online from three reputable websites that cover most of countries.

- **Amazon** - global online shopping retailer of everything
- **Biovea** - a global online retailer of high-end health products with a presence in many countries.
- **iHerb** - an international online store (including Korea, Japan, Spain, China & Russia), supplying a vast selection of brand name natural products. They now offer a very reasonable flat rate on international airmail. If you are ordering through iherb, use code NEX334 to get $5 off you order.

ACTION Strategise your "preventative supplement plan".

1. Identify your likely side effects and what supplements can you take proactively to minimise your risk.

2. Go to **www.managesideeffectsofchemo.com** for links to each of the online supplements companies.
-or-
 Email me via the **www.managesideeffectsofchemo.com** and request the list of links for all products in the following table.

3. Go online and purchase your supplements.

4.Prepare your first aid kit of natural supplements appropriate for your treatment phases.

SUPPLEMENT	SIDE EFFECT	WHERE TO BUY ONLINE
5-HTP	Hot Flushes	Vital Nutrients 5-HTP (Amazon) Metabolic Maintenance 5-HTP (Amazon) BIOVEA – AUST NZ USA CANADA UK STH AFRICA INDIA
Acetyl-L-Carnitine	Neuropathy	Vital Nutrients Acetyl-L-Carnitine (Amazon) Metabolic Maintenance Acetyl-L-Carnitine BIOVEA –AUST NZ USA CANADA UK STH AFRICA INDIA
Aggressive skin hydration cream	Hand Foot Syndrome (PPE)	Topix Urix 40 Urea Cream (Amazon)
AHCC	Weak immune system/ Low white blood cell count	Advance Physician Formulas AHCC 500 mg, 60 Capsules (Amazon) NOW Foods Ahcc 100 per cent Pure Powder BIOVEA –AUST NZ USA CANADA UK STH AFRICA INDIA
Alpha Lipoic Acid	Neuropathy	Vital Nutrients Alpha Lipoic Acid (Amazon) Metabolic Maintenance Alpha Lipoic Acid BIOVEA –AUST NZ USA CANADA UK STH AFRICA INDIA

SUPPLEMENT	SIDE EFFECT	WHERE TO BUY ONLINE
Antiperspirant deodorant	Hand Foot Syndrome (PPE)	Tom's of Maine (Natural) Antiperspirant Deodorant (Amazon) Ban Roll-On (unscented) Antiperspirant Deodorant (Amazon)
Astragalus	Fatigue (Stress)/ Weak immune system/ Organ damage	Gaia Herbs Astragalus(Amazon) Herb Pharm Astragalus (Amazon) Vital Nutrients Astragalus (Amazon) BIOVEA –AUST NZ USA CANADA UK STH AFRICA INDIA
B Vitamins	Fatigue	Vital Nutrients B-Complex 120 Capsules Metabolic Maintenance B-complex Vitamins BIOVEA –AUST NZ USA CANADA UK STH AFRICA INDIA
Bacopa	Brain fog/ memory loss	Herb Pharm Bacopa (Amazon) Thorne Bacopa
Berberine	Damage to intestines	Vital Nutrients Berberine(Amazon) Thorne Berberine (iherb)
Beta Glucan	Weak immune system	Beta Glucan (Amazon) Source Naturals Beta Glucan (iherb) BIOVEA –AUST NZ USA CANADA UK STH AFRICA INDIA
Bioflavonoids	Healing/ Cell damage/enhance radiation effect	Country Life Citrus Bioflavonoid Complex 1000 mg(Amazon) Solgar - Citrus Bioflavonoid Complex, 1000 mg (Amazon) Vital Nutrients Bioflavonoids (Amazon)
Black Cohosh	Hot Flushes	Gaia Herbs Black Cohosh (Amazon) Herb Pharm Black Cohosh (Amazon) BIOVEA –AUST NZ USA CANADA UK STH AFRICA INDIA

127

SUPPLEMENT	SIDE EFFECT	WHERE TO BUY ONLINE
Boswelia	Brain swelling	Boswelia (Amazon) BIOVEA –AUST NZ USA CANADA UK STH AFRICA INDIA
Bromelain	Healing/ Joint pain	Source Naturals Bromelain (iherb) Thorne Bromelain (iherb) Vital Nutrients Bromelain (Amazon) Metabolic Maintenance Bromelain (Amazon)
Calcium	Weak bone/risk of fracture/ Hair and nail health	Vital Nutrients Calcium (citrate/malate) 150 mg 100 capsules (Amazon) BIOVEA –AUST NZ USA CANADA UK STH AFRICA INDIA
Calendula lotion	Skin reactions	Herb Pharm Calendula (Amazon) Iherb Calendula Spray (iherb) Iherb cream (iherb)
Cat's Claw	Weak immune system	BIOVEA –AUST NZ USA CANADA UK STH AFRICA INDIA Iherb – Cats Claw (iherb)
Charcoal capsules	Diarrhea	Charcoal Capsules (Amazon) Iherb Charcoal Activated (iherb)
Coconut Oil	Skin reactions	Buy extra virgin, cold pressed, certified organic coconut oil form your local health food shop. Guide to buying coconut oil. Cert Organic Extra Virgin Coconut Oil (Amazon) Iherb Coconut Oil (iherb)
Cooling Gel Cap	Hair and nail health	Refer to your oncologist

SUPPLEMENT	SIDE EFFECT	WHERE TO BUY ONLINE
CoQ10	Cardiotoxicity, fatigue/ Fatigue	Vital Nutrients CoQ10(Amazon) Metabolic Maintenance CoQ10 (Amazon) BIOVEA –AUST NZ USA CANADA UK STH AFRICA INDIA Iherb CoQ10
Curcumin	Joint pain/ Inflammation/ enhance radiation effect	Vital Nutrients Curcumin(Amazon) BIOVEA –AUST NZ USA CANADA UK Iherb – Curcumin
DGL	Mouth sores	Vital Nutrients DGL(Amazon) BIOVEA –AUST NZ USA CANADA UK Iherb – DGL
Echinacea	Weak immune system	Herb Pharm Echinacea (iherb) Vital Nutrients Echinacea(Amazon) BIOVEA –AUST NZ USA CANADA UK STH AFRICA INDIA
Essential Fatty Acids (Omega 3/6)	Hair and nail health/ Inflammation/ enhance radiation effect/ Weak bone/risk of fracture	Krill Oil - superior form of Omega-3s Chia Seeds – highest plant source of Omega-3 known BIOVEA –AUST NZ USA CANADA UK STH AFRICA INDIA **Here are some foods that contain EFA:** Avocado, Almonds, Black current oil, Borage oil, Canola, Cashews, Dark green leaves, Evening primrose oil, Filberts (hazelnuts), Flax seed, Flax Oil, Flax Meal, Hemp seed oil, Macadamia Nuts, Olives, Peanuts and peanut oil, Pecans, Pumpkin oil, Safflower oil, Salmon, Sardines, Sesame seeds, Sesame oil, Soybeans, Sunflower seeds/oil, Tuna, Walnuts and purslane
Genistein /Soy Protein/ Isoflavones	Hot Flushes	Soy Protein(Amazon) Vital Nutrients – Genistein (80 per cent Soy Isoflavones) (Amazon) Genistein/Soy Isoflavones BIOVEA –AUST NZ USA CANADA UK Iherb – Soy Protein/Isoflavones/Geinistein

SUPPLEMENT	SIDE EFFECT	WHERE TO BUY ONLINE
Ginkgo biloba extract	DNA damage	Gaia Herbs Ginkgo Biloba Extract (Amazon) Herb Pharm Ginkgo Biloba (Amazon) Vital Nutrients Ginkgo Extract(Amazon) BIOVEA –AUST NZ USA CANADA UK STH AFRICA INDIA Iherb- Ginkgo Biloba
Glucosamine & Chondroitin	Joint pain	Vital Nutrients Glucosamine & Chondroitin Metabolic Maintenance Glucosamine & Chondroitin(Amazon) BIOVEA –AUST NZ USA CANADA UK STH AFRICA INDIA
Henna	Hand Foot Syndrome (PPE)	Henna (Amazon)
Hesperidin	Hot Flushes	Iherb – Hesperidin Pure Encapsulations Hesperidin Plus (Amazon) Thorne Research – HMC Hesperidin – 60's
Homeopathic Arnica	Reducing pain, swelling and bruising	Boiron Homeopathic Arnica (Amazon) BIOVEA –AUST NZ USA CANADA UK STH AFRICA INDIA Iherb – homeppathic Arnica
Homeopathic Eupatorium	Low white blood cell count/ Bone pain	Boiron Homeopathic Eupatorium (Amazon)
Homeopathic Gelsemium	Emotional support	Boiron Homeopathic Gelsemium(Amazon) BIOVEA –AUST NZ USA CANADA UK STH AFRICA INDIA Iherb – Homeopathic Gelsemium
Homeopathic Phosphorus	Emotional support/ Low white blood cell count	Boiron Homeopathic Phosphorus (Amazon) BIOVEA –AUST NZ USA CANADA UK STH AFRICA INDIA
Honey	Mouth sores/ Radiation induced mucositis	Manuka Honey(Amazon) Pure & natural honey if you cannot access Manuka Honey
Horsetail	Hair and nail health	Gaia Herbs Horsetail (Amazon) Herb Pharm Horsetail (Amazon) Iherb – Horsetail

SUPPLEMENT	SIDE EFFECT	WHERE TO BUY ONLINE
Inositol	Insomnia	Vital Nutrients Inositol (Amazon) BIOVEA –AUST NZ USA CANADA UK STH AFRICA INDIA Iherb – Inositol
L-Carnitine	Cardiotoxicity, fatigue/ Fatigue	Metabolic Maintenance – L- Carnitine 250mg 60 caps (Amazon) Iherb – L-Carnitine BIOVEA –AUST NZ USA CANADA UK STH AFRICA INDIA Note: L-Caritine is unable to be imported into Canada.
L-Glutamine	Diarrhea/ Mouth sores/ Neuropathy/ Irritated digestive tract	Metabolic Maintenance L-Glutamine (Amazon) BIOVEA –AUST NZ USA CANADA UK STH AFRICA INDIA Iherb – L-Glutamine
Magnesium/ Magnesium Citrate	Hot Flushes/ Weak bone/risk of fracture/ Hair and nail health/ Constipation	Vital Nutrients Magnesium Citrate (Amazon) Vital Nutrients Magnesium (Amazon) BIOVEA –AUST NZ USA CANADA UK STH AFRICA INDIA
Maitake	Weak immune system	Gaia Herbs Maitake (Amazon) Reishi Shiitake Maitake Mushroom Extract Iherb – Maitake
Melatonin	Insomnia	Vital Nutrients Melatonin (Amazon) Metabolic Maintenance Melatonin (Amazon) Iherb – Melotonin BIOVEA –AUST NZ USA CANADA UK STH AFRICA INDIA Note: Melatoin is prescription only in NZ. Suggest buy from Aust.
Mistletoe	Weak immune system	Herb Pharm Mistletoe (Amazon) Iherb – Mistletoe Mistletoe injections (Helixor& Iscador) available only through physicians
Modified Citrus Pectin (MCP)	Reducing the spread of cancer cells –metastasis	Vital Nutrients MCP (Modified Citrus Pectin) 360g (Amazon) Iherb – MCP
MSM	Joint pain	Vital Nutrients MSM (Amazon) BIOVEA –AUST NZ USA CANADA UK STH AFRICA INDIA Iherb – MSM

131

SUPPLEMENT	SIDE EFFECT	WHERE TO BUY ONLINE
Niacin	Enhance radiation effectiveness	Vital Nutrients – Niacin 500mg Extended Release 90t (Amazon) BIOVEA –AUST NZ USA CANADA UK STH AFRICA INDIA Iherb – Niacin
Papaya Leaf	Low white blood cell count	Papaya Leaf (Amazon)
Probiotics	Constipation/ Diarrhea	Thorne Research –Bacillus Coagulans (formerly Lactobacillus Sporogenes) (Amazon) Lactobacillus Acidophilus Probiotic Powder 15 Billion (Amazon) Benebiotics 18-strain Multi-probiotic Supplement with Lactobacillus Acidophilus, Bifidobacterium Infantis, Saccaharomyces Boulardii, and Prebiotic (Amazon) Iherb – probiotics
Quercetin	Cell damage/enhance radiation effect	Quercetin (Amazon) Iherb – Quercetin
Reishi	Weak immune system	Gaia Herbs Reishi (Amazon) Reishi Shiitake Maitake Mushroom Extract BIOVEA –AUST NZ USA CANADA UK STH AFRICA INDIA Iherb – Reishi
Rescue Remedy	Emotional support	Bach Flower Essences Rescue Remedy (Amazon)
Rhodiola Rosea	Fatigue (Stress)	Gaia Herbs Rhodiola Rosea (Amazon) Herb Pharm Rhodiola Rosea (Amazon) Vital Nutrients Rhodiola Rosea (Amazon) BIOVEA –AUST NZ USA CANADA UK STH AFRICA INDIA Iherb – Rhodiola Rosea

132

SUPPLEMENT	SIDE EFFECT	WHERE TO BUY ONLINE
Saw Palmetto	Urinary symptoms	Gaia Herbs Saw Palmetto (Amazon) Herb Pharm Saw Palmetto (Amazon) Vital Nutrients Saw Palmetto (Amazon) BIOVEA –AUST NZ USA CANADA UK STH AFRICA INDIA Iherb – Saw Palmetto
Sesame oil	Low white blood cell count	Buy extra virgin, cold pressed, certified organic coconut oil form your local health food shop
Shitake	Weak immune system	Mushroom Shitake Powder (Amazon) Reishi Shiitake Maitake Mushroom Extract Iherb –Shitake
Slippery Elm Bark	Urinary tract irritation	Gaia Herbs Slippery Elm Bark (Amazon) Vital Nutrients Slippery Elm Bark (Amazon) Iherb – Slippery Elm Bark
Soy Protein/ Genistein/ Isoflavones	Hot Flushes	Soy Protein (Amazon) Vital Nutrients - Genistein (80 per cent Soy Isoflavones) (Amazon) Genistein/Soy Isoflavones BIOVEA –AUST NZ USA CANADA UK Iherb – Soy Protein/Isoflavones/Geinistein
St. John's Wort	Weak immune system	Nature's Way St. John's Wort Capsules Yogi St. John's Wort Herbal Tea (Amazon) BIOVEA –AUST NZ USA CANADA UK STH AFRICA INDIA
Taurine	Cardiotoxicity, fatigue	Vital Nutrients Taurine (Amazon) Metabolic Maintenance Taurine (Amazon) BIOVEA –AUST NZ USA CANADA UK STH AFRICA INDIA Iherb - Taurine
Theanine	Insomnia	Vital Nutrients Theanine (Amazon) BIOVEA –AUST NZ USA CANADA UK STH AFRICA INDIA Iherb - Theanine

133

SUPPLEMENT	SIDE EFFECT	WHERE TO BUY ONLINE
Topical DMSO	Hand Foot Syndrome (PPE)	See your local compounding pharmacist to prepare a DMSO lotion of 99 per cent strength
Vitamin A	Proctitis	Vital Nutrients Vitamin A (Amazon)
Vitamin B6 (Pyridoxal Phosphate-PLP)	Neuropathy/ Hand Foot Syndrome (PPE)	Vital Nutrients Vitamin B6 (Amazon) Metabolic Maintenance Pyridoxal 5 Phosphate 100 caps (Amazon) BIOVEA –AUST NZ USA CANADA UK STH AFRICA INDIA
Vitamin C	Healing/ Hot Flushes	Vital Nutrients Vitamin C (Amazon) Metabolic Maintenance Vitamin C (Amazon) BIOVEA –AUST NZ USA CANADA UK STH AFRICA INDIA
Vitamin D	Weak bone/risk of fracture	Metabolic Maintenance Vitamin D3 (Amazon) NOW Foods Vitamin D3 (Amazon)
Zinc	Healing/ Hair and nail health	Vital Nutrients Zinc (Amazon) BIOVEA –AUST USA CANADA UK STH AFRICA INDIA

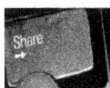

References Cited

[1] http://www.cancer.gov/cancertopics/factsheet/Sites-Types/metastatic
[2] Taylor A, Powell ME. Intensity-modulated radiotherapy—what is it? *Cancer Imaging* ; 4(2):68–73, 2004
[3] EFSA Panel on Dietetic Products, Nutrition, and Allergies (NDA). Scientific Opinion on Dietary Reference Values for Water. EFSA Journal, ;8(3):1459, 2010
[4] Guarner F, Malagelada JR. "Gut flora in health and disease". *Lancet* 361 (9356): 512–9, 2003
[5] Catenacci VA; Hill JO; Wyatt HR., The obesity epidemic. *Clin Chest Med* - 01-SEP-2009; 30(3): 415-44, vii.
[6] Reece EA., Perspectives on obesity, pregnancy and birth outcomes in the United States: the scope of the problem. - *Am J Obstet Gynecol* - 01-JAN-2008; 198(1): 23-7.
[7] Viera AJ; Sheridan SL., Global risk of coronary heart disease: assessment and application. *Am Fam Physician* - 1-AUG-2010; 82(3): 265-74.
[8] Chen L, Magliano DJ, Zimmet PZ. The worldwide epidemiology of type 2 diabetes mellitus-present and future perspectives. Nat Rev Endocrinol. 2011 Nov 8.
[9] Norton C, Georgiopoulou VV, Kalogeropoulos AP, Butler J. Epidemiology and cost of advanced heart failure. Prog Cardiovasc Dis. 2011 Sep-Oct;54(2):78-85
[10] Jenkins DJ; Sievenpiper JL; Pauly D; Sumaila UR; Kendall CW; Mowat FM., Are dietary recommendations for the use of fish oils sustainable? *CMAJ* - 17-MAR-2009; 180(6): 633-7
[11] Kilfoy BA; Zhang Y; Park Y; Holford TR; Schatzkin A; Hollenbeck A; Ward MH., Dietary nitrate and nitrite and the risk of thyroid cancer in the NIH-AARP Diet and Health Study. *Int J Cancer* - 1-JUL-2011; 129(1): 160-72.
[12] http://nutritiondata.self.com/foods-00006700000000000000.html
[13] http://www.hsph.harvard.edu/nutritionsource/what-should-you-eat/omega-3-fats/?__utma=1.1019172037.1330889662.1330889662.1330889662.1&__utmb=1.1.10.1330889662&__utmc=1&__utmx=-&__utmz=1.1330889662.1.1.utmcsr=hsph.harvard.edu|utmccn=(referral)|utmcmd=referral|utmcct=/&__utmv=-&__utmk=137737904
[14] Simopoulos AP., Evolutionary aspects of diet, the Omega-6/Omega-3 ratio and genetic variation: nutritional implications for chronic diseases. *Biomed Pharmacother* - 01-NOV-2006; 60(9): 502-7

[15] Harris W., Omega-6 and Omega-3 fatty acids: partners in prevention. *Curr Opin Clin Nutr Metab Care* - 01-MAR-2010; 13(2): 125-9

[16] Simopoulos AP The importance of the Omega-6/Omega-3 fatty acid ratio in cardiovascular disease and other chronic diseases. *Exp Biol Med (Maywood)* - 01-JUN-2008; 233(6): 674-88

[17] O'Keefe JH Jr, Cordain L., Cardiovascular disease resulting from a diet and lifestyle at odds with our Paleolithic genome: how to become a 21st-century hunter-gatherer., Mayo Clin Proc. 2004 Jan;79(1):101-8.

[18] Collino, M., High dietary fructose intake: Sweet or bitter life? World J Diabetes. 2011 Jun 15;2(6):77-81.

[19] Bray GA, Nielsen SJ, Popkin BM. Consumption of high-fructose corn syrup in beverages may play a role in the epidemic of obesity. Am J Clin Nutr. 2004 Apr;79(4):537-43.

[20] Moeller SM, Fryhofer SA, Osbaht, AJ, RobinowitzkmCB, Council on Science and Public Health, American Medical Association. *Et al*, The effects of high fructose syrup. J Am Coll Nutr. 2009 Dec;28(6):619-26.

[21] http://courses.swinburne.edu.au/subjects/Introduction-to-Mind%2FBody-Medicine-HIM205/local. (Accessed 6/2010)

[22] http://www.aima.net.au/resources/what_is_integrative_medicine.html (Accessed 6/2010)

[23] Friedman, HS, (2008) The Multiple Linkages of Personality and Disease, *Brain, Behavior, and Immunity,* 22(5):668–675.

[24] Irwin, MR,(2008) Human psychoneuroimmunology: 20 Years of Discovery, *Brain, Behavior, and Immunity, 22*, (2): 129-139.

[25] Goncharova, LB, Tarakanov, AO, (2007) Molecular Networks of Brain and Immunity, *Brain Research Reviews, 55,* (1):155-166.

[26] Malarkey, WB, Mills, PJ, (2007) Endocrinology: The active partner in PNI Research, *Brain, Behavior, and Immunity, 21(2):*161-168.

[27] Miller, RL, Ho, SM., (2008) Environmental epigenetics and asthma: current concepts and call for studies, *Am J Resp CritCareMed*(6):567-73.

[28] Epel ES, Blackburn EH, Lin J, Dhabhar FS, Adler NE, Morrow JD, Cawthon RM. (2004) Accelerated telomere shortening in response to life stress. *Proc Natl Acad Sci* U S A. Dec 7;101(49):17312-5.

[29] Macnee W., (2007) Pathogenesis of Chronic Obstructive Pulmonary Disease, *Clin Chest Med, 28*(3): 479-513, v.

[30] Taïeb, A., Hanifin,J., Cooper, K., Bos, JD, Imokawa, G., David, TJ.,*et al* (2006)Proceedings of the 4th Georg Rajka International Symposium on Atopic Dermatitis, Arcachon, France, September 15-17, , *J Allergy Clin Immunol* 117(2): 378-90, 2006.

[31] Fleming JL; Huang TH; Toland AE., (2008) The role of parental and grandparental epigenetic alterations in familial cancer risk. *Cancer Res*; 68(22): 9116-21.

[32] Mathews LA; Crea F; Farrar WL. (2009) Epigenetic gene regulation in stem cells and correlation to cancer.

Differentiation; 78(1): 1-17.

[33] Iacobuzio-Donahue CA. (2009) Epigenetic changes in cancer. *Annu Rev Pathol* 4: 229-49.

[34] Clark SJ., (2007) Action at a distance: epigenetic silencing of large chromosomal regions in carcinogenesis. *Hum Mol Genet* Spec No 1: R88-95.

[35] Weidman JR; Dolinoy DC; Murphy SK; Jirtle RL. (2007) Cancer susceptibility: epigenetic manifestation of environmental exposures. *Cancer J*; 13(1): 9-16.

[36] Hitchler MJ; Domann FE. (2009) Metabolic defects provide a spark for the epigenetic switch in cancer.
Free Radic Biol Med; 47(2): 115-27.

[37] Davis CD (2007) Nutritional interactions: credentialing of molecular targets for cancer prevention. *Exp Biol Med (Maywood)*; 232(2): 176-83.

[38] Dutkiewicz MC.,(2008) - Lifting a fork to heart health. Whole foods as a treatment intervention. *Adv Nurse Pract*; 16(2): 57-60

[39] Ross SA (2007) Nutritional genomic approaches to cancer prevention research. *Exp Oncol*; 29(4): 250-6.

[40] Herceg Z., (2007) Epigenetics and cancer: towards an evaluation of the impact of environmental and dietary factors. *Mutagenesis*; 22(2): 91-103.

[41].Choudhuri S (2010) Molecular targets of epigenetic regulation and effectors of environmental influences *Toxicol Appl Pharmacol*; 245(3): 378-93

[42] Nystrom M.,(2009) Diet and epigenetics in colon cancer. *World J Gastroenterol*; 15(3): 257-63.

[43] Feinberg AP, (2004) The epigenetics of cancer etiology. *Semin Cancer Biol,* 14(6): 427-32.

[44] Herceg Z, Vaissière T. Epigenetic mechanisms and **cancer**: an interface between the environment and the genome. Epigenetics. 2011 Jul;6(7):804-19.

[45] Lujambio A; Esteller M., (2009) How epigenetics can explain human metastasis: a new role for microRNAs. *Cell Cycle*; 8(3): 377-82

[46] Feinberg AP., (2007) Phenotypic plasticity and the epigenetics of human disease. *Nature*; 447(7143): 433-40

[47] Ege MJ, Bieli, C., van Strien, RT, Riedler, J., Ublagger, E, Schram-Bijkerk, D *et al* (2006) Prenatal Farm Exposure is Related to the Expression of Receptors of the Innate Immunity and to atopic sensitization in school-age children, *J Allergy Clin Immunol*; 117(4): 817-23.

[48] Vercelli, D., (2004) Genetics, epigenetics, and the environment: switching, buffering, releasing. *J. Allergy Clin Immunol*;*113*(3):381-6.

[49] Waterland RA , (2006) Epigenetic Mechanisms and Gastrointestinal Development- *J Pediatr* ; 149(5 Suppl); S137-S142.

[50] Trujillo E, Davis, C., Milner, J. (2006) Nutrigenomics, proteomics, metabolomics and the practice of dietetics, *J Am Diet Assoc*; *106*(3): 403-

13.

[51] Reynolds E, (2006) Vitamin B12, folic acid, and the nervous system, *Lancet Neurol*; 5(11): 949-60.

[52] Macnee W, (2007) Pathogenesis of Chronic Obstructive Pulmonary Disease, *Clin Chest Med* , 28(3): 479-513, v.

[53] Herzeg, Z., (2007) Epigenetics and Cancer: Towards an evaluation of the impact of environmental and dietary factors, *Mutagenesis*, 22(2), 91-103.

[54] Crews, D., (2008) Epigenetics and its implications for behavioral neuroendocrinology, *Frontiers in Neuroendocrinology, 29(3)*, 344-357.

[55] Yoo GJ; Aviv C; Levine EG; Ewing C; Au A, (2010) Emotion work: disclosing cancer. *Support Care Cancer,* 18(2): 205-15

[56] Kreuter MW *et al (*2008) What makes cancer survivor stories work? An empirical study among African American women. - *J Cancer Surviv-*; 2(1): 33-44.

[57] Eliott JA; Olver IN (2007) Hope and hoping in the talk of dying cancer patients. *Soc Sci Med* , 64(1): 138-49.

[58] Schroevers M; Kraaij V; Garnefski N, (2008) How do cancer patients manage unattainable personal goals and regulate their emotions? *Br J Health Psychol*; 13(Pt 3): 551-62

[59] Meyerowitz BE; Kurita K; D'Orazio LM, (2008) The psychological and emotional fallout of cancer and its treatment. *Cancer J*; 14(6): 410-3

[60] Desiere, F. (2004) Towards a systems biology understanding of human health: Interplay between genotype, environment and nutrition, *Biotechnology Annual Review,* 10:51-84.

[61] Ornish, D., Magbanua MJ, Weidner G, Weinberg V, Kemp C, Green C, Mattie MD, Marlin R, Simko J, Shinohara K, Haqq CM, Carroll PR , (2008) Changes in prostate gene expression in men undergoing an intensive nutrition and lifestyle intervention., *PNAS, 105(24):*8369-74, (Epub) .

[62] Prasad AS. Zinc and immunity. *Mol Cell Biochem.* 1998 Nov;188(1-2):63-9. http://www.ncbi.nlm.nih.gov/pubmed/9823012?dopt=Abstract

[63] Nathens AB, Neff MJ, Jurkovich GJ, Klotz P, Farver K, Ruzinski JT, Radella F, Garcia I, Maier RV. Randomised, prospective trial of antioxidant supplementation in critically ill surgical patients. *Ann Surg.* 2002 Dec;236(6):814-22.   http://www.ncbi.nlm.nih.gov/pubmed/12454520

[64] Coleridge-Smith P, Lok C, Ramelet AA. Venous leg ulcer: a meta-analysis of adjunctive therapy with micronised purified flavonoid fraction. *Eur J Vasc Endovasc Surg.* 2005 Aug;30(2):198-208. http://www.ncbi.nlm.nih.gov/pubmed/15936227

[65] Onken JE, Greer PK, Calingaert B, Hale LP. Bromelain treatment decreases secretion of pro-inflammatory cytokines and chemokines by colon biopsies in vitro. *Clin Immunol.* 2008 Mar;126(3):345-52. Epub 2007 Dec 21.   http://www.ncbi.nlm.nih.gov/pubmed/18160345

[66] Glinsky VV, Raz A. Modified citrus pectin anti-metastatic properties: one bullet, multiple targets. *Carbohydr Res.* 2009 Sep 28;344(14):1788-91.

Epub 2008 Sep 26. http://www.ncbi.nlm.nih.gov/pubmed/19061992

[67] Guess BW, Scholz MC, Strum SB, Lam RY, Johnson HJ, Jennrich RI. Modified citrus pectin (MCP) increases the prostate-specific antigen doubling time in men with prostate cancer: a phase II pilot study. *Prostate Cancer Prostatic Dis.* 2003;6(4):301-4. http://www.ncbi.nlm.nih.gov/pubmed/14663471

[68] Platt D, Raz A. Modulation of the lung colonisation of B16-F1 melanoma cells by citrus pectin. *J Natl Cancer Inst.* 1992 Mar 18;84(6):438-42. http://www.ncbi.nlm.nih.gov/pubmed/1538421

[69] Homeopathy. 2007 Jan;96(1):17-21. Homeopathic Arnica montana for post-tonsillectomy analgesia: a randomised placebo control trial. Robertson A, Suryanarayanan R, Banerjee A. http://www.ncbi.nlm.nih.gov/pubmed/17227743

[70] Arch Facial Plast Surg. 2006 Jan-Feb;8(1):54-9. Effect of homeopathic Arnica montana on bruising in face-lifts: results of a randomised, double-blind, placebo-controlled clinical trial. Seeley BM, Denton AB, Ahn MS, Maas CS. http://www.ncbi.nlm.nih.gov/pubmed/16415448

[71] Healing With Bach® Flower Essences: Testing a Complementary Therapy. Complementary Health Practice Review January 2007 12: 3-14, Halberstein R, DeSantis L, and Sirkin A. http://chp.sagepub.com/content/12/1/3.abstract

[72] Integr Cancer Ther. 2005 Jun;4(2):110-30. Coenzyme q10 for prevention of anthracycline-induced cardiotoxicity. Conklin KA. http://www.ncbi.nlm.nih.gov/pubmed/15911925

[73] J Cancer Res Clin Oncol. 2006 Feb;132(2):121-8. Epub 2005 Nov 8. Effects of doxorubicin-containing chemotherapy and a combination with L-carnitine on oxidative metabolism in patients with non-Hodgkin lymphoma. Waldner R, Laschan C, Lohninger A, Gessner M, Tüchler H, Huemer M, Spiegel W, Karlic H. http://www.ncbi.nlm.nih.gov/pubmed/16283381

[74] Adv Exp Med Biol. 2009;643:65-74. Beneficial effect of taurine treatment against doxorubicin-induced cardiotoxicity in mice. Ito T, Muraoka S, Takahashi K, Fujio Y, Schaffer SW, Azuma J. http://www.ncbi.nlm.nih.gov/pubmed/19239137

[75] Eur J Clin Nutr. 2003 Dec;57 Suppl 2:S88-95. Mild dehydration: a risk factor of constipation? Arnaud MJ. http://www.ncbi.nlm.nih.gov/pubmed/14681719

[76] J Pediatr (Rio J). 2011 Jan-Feb;87(1):24-8. Epub 2010 Nov 29. Comparison of the effectiveness of polyethylene glycol 4000 without electrolytes and magnesium hydroxide in the treatment of chronic functional constipation in children. Gomes PB, Duarte MA, Melo Mdo C. http://www.ncbi.nlm.nih.gov/pubmed/21116598

[77] J Clin Gastroenterol. 2010 Sep;44 Suppl 1:S30-4. The use of probiotics in healthy volunteers with evacuation disorders and hard stools: a double-blind, randomised, placebo-controlled study. Del Piano M, Carmagnola S,

Anderloni A, Andorno S, Ballarè M, Balzarini M, Montino F, Orsello M, Pagliarulo M, Sartori M, Tari R, Sforza F, Capurso L.
http://www.ncbi.nlm.nih.gov/pubmed/20697291
[78] Aliment Pharmacol Ther. 2009 Sep 1;30(5):452-8. Epub 2009 Jun 15. Clinical trial: prophylactic intravenous alanyl-glutamine reduces the severity of gastrointestinal toxicity induced by chemotherapy--a randomised crossover study. Li Y, Ping X, Yu B, Liu F, Ni X, Li J.
http://www.ncbi.nlm.nih.gov/pubmed/19549287
[79] Ann Trop Paediatr. 2010;30(4):299-304. Lactobacillus acidophilus and Bifidobacterium bifidum stored at ambient temperature are effective in the treatment of acute diarrhoea. Rerksuppaphol S, Rerksuppaphol L.
http://www.ncbi.nlm.nih.gov/pubmed/21118623
[80] American Family Physician. 2008, 78(9):1073-8 Probiotics. Kligler B, Cohrssen A.

http://ukpmc.ac.uk/abstract/MED/19007054/reload=0;jsessionid=LMyGEF
dA48FC88KMcdWf.80
[81] J Clin Oncol. 2004 Nov 1;22(21):4410-7. Phase II study of activated charcoal to prevent irinotecan-induced diarrhea. Michael M, Brittain M, Nagai J, Feld R, Hedley D, Oza A, Siu L, Moore MJ.
http://www.ncbi.nlm.nih.gov/pubmed/15514383
[82] J Pain Symptom Manage. 2006 Dec;32(6):551-9. Safety, tolerability and symptom outcomes associated with L-carnitine supplementation in patients with cancer, fatigue, and carnitine deficiency: a phase I/II study. Cruciani RA, Dvorkin E, Homel P, Malamud S, Culliney B, Lapin J, Portenoy RK, Esteban-Cruciani N.
http://www.ncbi.nlm.nih.gov/pubmed/17157757
[83] MMW Fortschr Med. 2008 Jan 17;149 Suppl 4:162-6. [Efficacy of a combination therapy with vitamins B6, B12 and folic acid for general feeling of ill-health. Results of a non-interventional post-marketing surveillance study]. Engels A, Schröer U, Schremmer D.
http://www.ncbi.nlm.nih.gov/pubmed/18402241
[84] Nutrition. 2010 Mar;26(3):250-4. Epub 2009 Nov 22. Clinical aspects of coenzyme Q10: an update.
Littarru GP, Tiano L. http://www.ncbi.nlm.nih.gov/pubmed/19932599
[85] Planta Med. 2009 Feb;75(2):105-12. Epub 2008 Nov 18. A randomised, double-blind, placebo-controlled, parallel-group study of the standardised extract shr-5 of the roots of Rhodiola rosea in the treatment of subjects with stress-related fatigue. Olsson EM, von Schéele B, Panossian AG.
http://www.ncbi.nlm.nih.gov/pubmed/19016404
[86] Zhongguo Zhong Xi Yi Jie He Za Zhi. 2003 Oct;23(10):733-5. Effect of astragalus injection combined with chemotherapy on quality of life in patients with advanced non-small cell lung cancer. Zou YH, Liu XM.
http://www.ncbi.nlm.nih.gov/pubmed/14626183

[87] Breast Cancer. 2010 Oct;17(4):298-302. Epub 2009 Sep 30. Impact of prophylactic pyridoxine on occurrence of hand-foot syndrome in patients receiving capecitabine for advanced or metastatic breast cancer. Yoshimoto N, Yamashita T, Fujita T, Hayashi H, Tsunoda N, Kimura M, Tsuzuki N, Yamashita H, Toyama T, Kondo N, Iwata H.
http://www.ncbi.nlm.nih.gov/pubmed/19789949

[88] Invest New Drugs. 2008 Apr;26(2):189-92. Epub 2007 Sep 21. Topical henna for capecitabine induced hand-foot syndrome. Yucel I, Guzin G.
http://www.ncbi.nlm.nih.gov/pubmed?term=henna
capecitabine&cmd=correctspelling

[89] Cancer Chemother Pharmacol. 1999;44(4):303-6. Topical DMSO treatment for pegylated liposomal doxorubicin-induced palmar-plantar erythrodysesthesia. Lopez AM, Wallace L, Dorr RT, Koff M, Hersh EM, Alberts DS. http://www.ncbi.nlm.nih.gov/pubmed/10447577

[90] Altern Ther Health Med. 2010 Jan-Feb;16(1):36-44. Efficacy of black cohosh-containing preparations on menopausal symptoms: a meta-analysis. Shams T, Setia MS, Hemmings R, McCusker J, Sewitch M, Ciampi A.
http://www.ncbi.nlm.nih.gov/pubmed/20085176

[91] Nutr Cancer. 2007;59(2):269-77. Black cohosh does not exert an estrogenic effect on the breast.
Ruhlen RL, Haubner J, Tracy JK, Zhu W, Ehya H, Lamberson WR, Rottinghaus GE, Sauter ER.
http://www.ncbi.nlm.nih.gov/pubmed/18001221

[92] Altern Med Rev. 2003 Aug;8(3):284-302. Hot flashes--a review of the literature on alternative and complementary treatment approaches. Philp HA. http://www.ncbi.nlm.nih.gov/pubmed/12946239

[93] Smith CJ. Non-hormonal control of vasomotor flushing in menopausal patients. Chic Med 1964;67:193-195.
http://www.ncbi.nlm.nih.gov/pubmed/14132222

[94] Altern Med Rev. 2005 Sep;10(3):216-21. The potential of 5-hydryoxytryptophan for hot flash reduction: a hypothesis. Curcio JJ, Kim LS, Wollner D, Pockaj BA.
http://www.ncbi.nlm.nih.gov/pubmed/16164376

[95] Breast Cancer Res Treat. 2011 Feb 2. Erratum to: Soy intake in association with menopausal symptoms during the first 6 and 36 months after breast cancer diagnosis.
http://www.ncbi.nlm.nih.gov/pubmed?term=Breast Cancer Res Treat. 2011 Feb
Dorjgochoo T, Gu K, Zheng Y, Kallianpur A, Chen Z, Zheng W, Lu W, Shu XO.

[96] JAMA. 2009 Dec 9;302(22):2437-43. Soy food intake and breast cancer survival. Shu XO, Zheng Y, Cai H, Gu K, Chen Z, Zheng W, Lu W.
http://www.ncbi.nlm.nih.gov/pubmed/19996398

[97] Support Care Cancer. 2011 Jun;19(6):859-63. Epub 2011 Jan 27. A pilot

phase II trial of magnesium supplements to reduce menopausal hot flashes in breast cancer patients. Park H, Parker GL, Boardman CH, Morris MM, Smith TJ. http://www.ncbi.nlm.nih.gov/pubmed/21271347

[98] Psychopharmacology (Berl). 2011 Jul;216(1):111-20. Epub 2011 Feb 22. Evaluation of sleep, puberty and mental health in children with long-term melatonin treatment for chronic idiopathic childhood sleep onset insomnia. http://www.ncbi.nlm.nih.gov/pubmed/21340475

[99] Biol Psychol. 2007 Jan;74(1):39-45. Epub 2006 Aug 22. L-Theanine reduces psychological and physiological stress responses. Kimura K, Ozeki M, Juneja LR, Ohira H. http://www.ncbi.nlm.nih.gov/pubmed/16930802

[100] J Clin Psychopharmacol. 2001 Jun;21(3):335-9. Double-blind, controlled, crossover trial of inositol versus fluvoxamine for the treatment of panic disorder. Palatnik A, Frolov K, Fux M, Benjamin J. http://www.ncbi.nlm.nih.gov/pubmed/11386498

[101] Clin Exp Rheumatol. 2006 Jan-Feb;24(1):25-30. Efficacy and tolerance of an oral enzyme combination in painful osteoarthritis of the hip. A double-blind, randomised study comparing oral enzymes with non-steroidal anti-inflammatory drugs. Klein G, Kullich W, Schnitker J, Schwann H. http://www.ncbi.nlm.nih.gov/pubmed?term=Efficacy and tolerance of an oral enzyme combination ..

[102] Cancer Causes Control. 2011 Sep;22(9):1333-42. Epub 2011 Jun 25. Use of glucosamine and chondroitin and lung cancer risk in the VITamins And Lifestyle (VITAL) cohort. Brasky TM, Lampe JW, Slatore CG, White E. http://www.ncbi.nlm.nih.gov/pubmed/21706174

[103] Osteoarthritis Cartilage. 2006 Mar;14(3):286-94. Epub 2005 Nov 23. Efficacy of methylsulfonylmethane (MSM) in osteoarthritis pain of the knee: a pilot clinical trial. Kim LS, Axelrod LJ, Howard P, Buratovich N, Waters RF. http://www.ncbi.nlm.nih.gov/pubmed/16309928

[104] Nat Prod Rep. 2011 Oct 6. Multitargeting by curcumin as revealed by molecular interaction studies. Gupta SC, Prasad S, Kim JH, Patchva S, Webb LJ, Priyadarsini IK, Aggarwal BB. http://www.ncbi.nlm.nih.gov/pubmed/21979811

[105] Surg Endosc. 2011 Jun 14. Efficacy of turmeric (curcumin) in pain and postoperative fatigue after laparoscopic cholecystectomy: a double-blind, randomised placebo-controlled study. Agarwal KA, Tripathi CD, Agarwal BB, Saluja S. http://www.ncbi.nlm.nih.gov/pubmed/21671126

[106] J Laryngol Otol. 2009 Feb;123(2):223-8. Epub 2008 May 19. Honey as topical prophylaxis against radiochemotherapy-induced mucositis in head and neck cancer. Rashad UM, Al-Gezawy SM, El-Gezawy E, Azzaz AN. http://www.ncbi.nlm.nih.gov/pubmed/18485252

[107] Int J Radiat Oncol Biol Phys. 2000 Feb 1;46(3):535-9. Oral glutamine to alleviate radiation-induced oral mucositis: a pilot randomised trial. Huang EY, Leung SW, Wang CJ, Chen HC, Sun LM, Fang FM, Yeh SA, Hsu HC, Hsiung CY. http://www.ncbi.nlm.nih.gov/pubmed/10701731

[108] Haematologica. 2003 Feb;88(2):192-200. Glutamine-enriched parenteral nutrition after autologous peripheral blood stem cell transplantation: effects on immune reconstitution and mucositis. Piccirillo N, De Matteis S, Laurenti L, Chiusolo P, Sorà F, Pittiruti M, Rutella S, Cicconi S, Fiorini A, D'Onofrio G, Leone G, Sica S.
http://www.ncbi.nlm.nih.gov/pubmed/12604409

[109] J Assoc Physicians India. 1989 Oct;37(10):647. Deglycyrrhizinated liquorice in aphthous ulcers. Das SK, Das V, Gulati AK, Singh VP.
http://www.ncbi.nlm.nih.gov/pubmed/2632514

[110] Indian J Pediatr. 2010 Jun;77(6):681-3. Epub 2010 Jun 8.Use of pyridoxine and pyridostigmine in children with vincristine-induced neuropathy. Akbayram S, Akgun C, Doğan M, Sayin R, Caksen H, Oner AF. http://www.ncbi.nlm.nih.gov/pubmed/20532679

[111] Clin Oncol (R Coll Radiol). 2005 Jun;17(4):271-6. Glutamine as a neuroprotective agent in high-dose paclitaxel-induced peripheral neuropathy: a clinical and electrophysiologic study. Stubblefield MD, Vahdat LT, Balmaceda CM, Troxel AB, Hesdorffer CS, Gooch CL.
http://www.ncbi.nlm.nih.gov/pubmed/15997923

[112] Ther Clin Risk Manag. 2011;7:377-85. Epub 2011 Sep 5. Critical appraisal of the use of alpha lipoic acid (thioctic acid) in the treatment of symptomatic diabetic polyneuropathy. McIlduff CE, Rutkove SB.
http://www.ncbi.nlm.nih.gov/pubmed/21941444

[113] CNS Drugs. 2007;21 Suppl 1:39-43; discussion 45-6. Acetyl-L-carnitine for the treatment of chemotherapy-induced peripheral neuropathy: a short review. De Grandis D. http://www.ncbi.nlm.nih.gov/pubmed/17696592

[114] Ned Tijdschr Geneeskd. 2011;155(45):A3768. Scalp cooling for chemotherapy- induced alopecia. Komen MM, Smorenburg CH, van den Hurk CJ, Nortier JW. http://www.ncbi.nlm.nih.gov/pubmed/22085565

[115] Bull Cancer. 2011 Oct 1;98(9):1119-29. doi: 10.1684/bdc.2011.1430. Effectiveness of scalp cooling in chemotherapy. Poder TG, He J, Lemieux R. http://www.ncbi.nlm.nih.gov/pubmed/21914579

[116]Serrano Fernández MP, Gutiérrez Vilella MJ, Pérez Martín-Palanco A, Vanaclocha Sebastián F, Cabezón Gutiérrez L.
Servicio de Dermatología del Hospital Universitario 12 de Octubre. Rev Enferm. 2011 Sep;34(9):42-6. Palmar-plantar erythrodysaesthesia syndrome local cold prevention http://www.ncbi.nlm.nih.gov/pubmed/22013712

[117] http://annonc.oxfordjournals.org/content/16/3/352.full

[118] Clin Dermatol. 2010 Jul-Aug;28(4):420-5. Nutrition and nail disease. Cashman MW, Sloan SB. http://www.ncbi.nlm.nih.gov/pubmed/20620759

[119] J Dermatol Sci. 2011 Dec;64(3):153-8. Epub 2011 Aug 22. Integral hair lipid in human hair follicle. Lee WS.
http://www.ncbi.nlm.nih.gov/pubmed/21906914

[120] Br Med Bull (1981) 37 (1): 59-64. Essential Fatty Acid Deficiency.
http://bmb.oxfordjournals.org/content/37/1/59.extract
[121] BMC Plant Biol. 2011 Jul 29;11:112 New insight into silica deposition in horsetail (Equisetum arvense). Law C, Exley C
http://www.ncbi.nlm.nih.gov/pubmed/21801378
[122] Bull Exp Biol Med. 2008 Apr;145(4):464-6. Evaluation of antitumor activity of peptide extracts from medicinal plants on the model of transplanted breast cancer in CBRB-Rb(8.17)1Iem mice. Tepkeeva II, Moiseeva EV, Chaadaeva AV, Zhavoronkova EV, Kessler YV, Semushina SG, Demushkin VP. http://www.ncbi.nlm.nih.gov/pubmed/19110595
[123] Arzneimittelforschung. 1981;31(4):732-6. A controlled clinical trial for testing the efficacy of the homeopathic drug eupatorium perfoliatum D2 inthe treatment of common cold. Gassinger CA, Wünstel G, Netter P.
http://www.ncbi.nlm.nih.gov/pubmed/7195723
[124] J Hepatol. 2002 Jul;37(1):78-86. Improved prognosis of postoperative hepatocellular carcinoma patients when treated with functional foods: a prospective cohort study. Matsui Y, Uhara J, Satoi S, Kaibori M, Yamada H, Kitade H, Imamura A, Takai S, Kawaguchi Y, Kwon AH, Kamiyama Y.
http://www.ncbi.nlm.nih.gov/pubmed?term=J Hepatol.
[125] Wien Klin Wochenschr. 2009 Oct;121 Suppl 3:19-22. Thrombocyte counts in mice after the administration of papaya leaf suspension. Sathasivam K, Ramanathan S, Mansor SM, Haris MR, Wernsdorfer WH.
http://www.ncbi.nlm.nih.gov/pubmed/19915811
[126] Fitoterapia. 2011 Apr;82(3):383-92. Epub 2010 Nov 12. Protective effect of flavonoids from Astragalus complanatus on radiation induced damages in mice. Qi L, Liu CY, Wu WQ, Gu ZL, Guo CY.
http://www.ncbi.nlm.nih.gov/pubmed/21075176
[127] Clin Cancer Res. 1997 Oct;3(10):1775-9. Flavonoids as enhancers of x-ray-induced cell damage in hepatoma cells.
van Rijn J, van den Berg J.
http://www.ncbi.nlm.nih.gov/pubmed/Flavonoids
[128] J Thorac Oncol. 2011 Apr;6(4):688-98. Soy isoflavones augment radiation effect by inhibiting APE1/Ref-1 DNA repair activity in non-small cell lung cancer. Singh-Gupta V, Joiner MC, Runyan L, Yunker CK, Sarkar FH, Miller S, Gadgeel SM, Konski AA, Hillman GG.
http://www.ncbi.nlm.nih.gov/pubmed/21325978
[129] Int J Radiat Oncol Biol Phys. 2011 Mar 15;79(4):1206-15. Epub 2011 Jan 13.
Curcumin regulates low-linear energy transfer γ-radiation-induced NFκB-dependent telomerase activity in human neuroblastoma cells. Aravindan N, Veeraraghavan J, Madhusoodhanan R, Herman TS, Natarajan M.
http://www.ncbi.nlm.nih.gov/pubmed/21236599
[130] Strahlenther Onkol. 2011 Feb;187(2):127-34. Epub 2011 Jan 18. Omega-3 fatty acid supplementation in cancer therapy : does eicosapentanoic acid

influence the radiosensitivity of tumor cells? Manda K, Kriesen S, Hildebrandt G, Fietkau R, Klautke G.
http://www.ncbi.nlm.nih.gov/pubmed/21267532
[131] J Clin Endocrinol Metab. 2007 Nov;92(11):4286-9. Epub 2007 Aug 21. Anticlastogenic effect of Ginkgo biloba extract in Graves' disease patients receiving radioiodine therapy. Dardano A, Ballardin M, Ferdeghini M, Lazzeri E, Traino C, Caraccio N, Mariani G, Barale R, Monzani F.
http://www.ncbi.nlm.nih.gov/pubmed/17711926
[132] Free Radic Biol Med. 1995 Jun;18(6):985-91. Radiation-induced clastogenic factors: anticlastogenic effect of Ginkgo biloba extract. Emerit I, Arutyunyan R, Oganesian N, Levy A, Cernjavsky L, Sarkisian T, Pogossian A, Asrian K. http://www.ncbi.nlm.nih.gov/pubmed/7628734
[133] Pol Merkur Lekarski. 2010 Jul;29(169):54-7. [The usefulness of nicotinamide in radioiodine therapy in patients with toxic and nontoxic large goitres]. Mojsak MN, Rogowski F.
http://www.ncbi.nlm.nih.gov/pubmed/The usefulness of nicotinamide in radioiodine therapy
[134] Semin Oncol Nurs. 2011 May;27(2):e1-17. Evidence-based skin care management in radiation therapy: clinical update. McQuestion M.
http://www.ncbi.nlm.nih.gov/pubmed/21514477
[135] Dermatitis. 2004 Sep;15(3):109-16. A randomised double-blind controlled trial comparing extra virgin coconut oil with mineral oil as a moisturizer for mild to moderate xerosis. Agero AL, Verallo-Rowell VM.
http://www.ncbi.nlm.nih.gov/pubmed/15724344
[136] Int J Oral Maxillofac Surg. 2010 Dec;39(12):1181-5. Epub 2010 Sep 15. Effect of topical honey on limitation of radiation-induced oral mucositis: an intervention study. Khanal B, Baliga M, Uppal N.
http://www.ncbi.nlm.nih.gov/pubmed/20832243
[137]Topkan E, Yavuz MN, Onal C, Yavuz AA. Prevention of acute radiation-induced esophagitis with glutamine in non-small cell lung cancer patients treated with radiotherapy: evaluation of clinical and dosimetric parameters. Lung Cancer. 2009 Mar;63(3):393-9. Epub 2008 Aug 8.
http://www.ncbi.nlm.nih.gov/pubmed/18691789
[138] Br J Clin Pharmacol. 1984 Sep;18(3):461-2. A double-blind trial of an extract of the plant Serenoa repens in benign prostatic hyperplasia.
http://www.ncbi.nlm.nih.gov/pubmed/6207850
Champault G, Patel JC, Bonnard AM.
[139] Cell Biol Int. 2001;25(11):1117-24. Saw palmetto berry extract inhibits cell growth and Cox-2 expression in prostatic cancer cells. Goldmann WH, Sharma AL, Currier SJ, Johnston PD, Rana A, Sharma CP.
http://www.ncbi.nlm.nih.gov/pubmed/11913955
[140] J Altern Complement Med. 2010 Oct;16(10):1065-71. Effects of two natural medicine formulations on irritable bowel syndrome symptoms: a pilot study. Hawrelak JA, Myers SP.

145

http://www.ncbi.nlm.nih.gov/pubmed/20954962
[141] PLoS One. 2011 Apr 6;6(4):e18625. Prediagnostic plasma vitamin D metabolites and mortality among patients with prostate cancer. Fang F, Kasperzyk JL, Shui I, Hendrickson W, Hollis BW, Fall K, Ma J, Gaziano JM, Stampfer MJ, Mucci LA, Giovannucci E.
http://www.ncbi.nlm.nih.gov/pubmed/21494639
[142] Acta Anaesthesiol Scand. 2009 Sep;53(8):1088-91. Epub 2009 Jun 10. Intravenous magnesium sulfate for post-operative pain in patients undergoing lower limb orthopedic surgery. Dabbagh A, Elyasi H, Razavi SS, Fathi M, Rajaei S. http://www.ncbi.nlm.nih.gov/pubmed/19519724
[143] MDI 301, a nonirritating retinoid, improves abrasion wound healing in damaged/atrophic skin
Roscoe L. Warner, Narasimharao Bhagavathula, Kamalakar Nerusu, Andrew Hanosh, Shannon D. McClintock, Madhav K. Naik, Kent J. Johnson, Isaac Ginsburg, James Varani. Wound Repair Regen. Author manuscript; available in PMC 2010 May
6.http://www.ncbi.nlm.nih.gov/pmc/articles/PMC2865232/?tool=pmcentrez
[144] Med Oncol. 2010 Sep;27(3):919-25. Epub 2009 Sep 16.
Berberine inhibits acute radiation intestinal syndrome in human with abdomen radiotherapy.
Li GH, Wang DL, Hu YD, Pu P, Li DZ, Wang WD, Zhu B, Hao P, Wang J, Xu XQ, Wan JQ, Zhou YB, Chen ZT.
http://www.ncbi.nlm.nih.gov/pubmed/19757213
[145] Cancer. 2011 Aug 15;117(16):3788-95. doi: 10.1002/cncr.25945. Epub 2011 Feb 1.
Boswellia serrata acts on cerebral edema in patients irradiated for brain tumors: a prospective, randomised, placebo-controlled, double-blind pilot trial. http://www.ncbi.nlm.nih.gov/pubmed/21287538
Kirste S, Treier M, Wehrle SJ, Becker G, Abdel-Tawab M, Gerbeth K, Hug MJ, Lubrich B, Grosu AL, Momm F.
[146] J Altern Complement Med. 2010 Jul;16(7):753-9. Does Bacopa monnieri improve memory performance in older persons? Results of a randomised, placebo-controlled, double-blind trial. Morgan A, Stevens J.
http://www.ncbi.nlm.nih.gov/pubmed/20590480
[147] [Effects of large dose of Astragalus membranaceus on the dendritic cell induction of peripheral mononuclear cell and antigen presenting ability of dendritic cells in children with acute leukemia]. Dong J, Gu HL, Ma CT, Zhang F, Chen Z, Zhang Y. Zhongguo Zhong Xi Yi Jie He Za Zhi. 2005 Oct;25(10):872-5. Chinese.
http://www.ncbi.nlm.nih.gov/pubmed/16313105
[148] Evid Based Complement Alternat Med. 2005 Sep;2(3):309-14.
Echinacea: a miracle herb against aging and cancer? Evidence in vivo in mice. Miller SC. http://www.ncbi.nlm.nih.gov/pubmed/16136209
[149] Arzneimittelforschung. 2008;58(11):592-7. Comparison of Viscum

album QuFrF extract with vincristine in an in vitro model of human B cell lymphoma WSU-1. Kovacs E, Link S, Toffol-Schmidt U.
http://www.ncbi.nlm.nih.gov/pubmed/19137911

[150] Shah, S. A., Sander, S., White, C. M., Rinaldi, M., and Coleman, C. I. Evaluation of echinacea for the prevention and treatment of the common cold: a meta-analysis. Lancet Infect.Dis 2007;7(7):473-480.

[151] Weng, X. S. Treatment of leucopenia with pure Astragalus preparation--an analysis of 115 leucopenic cases. Zhongguo Zhong.Xi.Yi.Jie.He.Za Zhi. 1995;15(8):462-464.

[152] Borchers, A. T., Stern, J. S., Hackman, R. M., Keen, C. L., and Gershwin, M. E. Mushrooms, tumors, and immunity. Proc Soc Exp Biol Med 1999;221(4):281-293.

[153] Arinaga, S., Karimine, N., Takamuku, K., Nanbara, S., Inoue, H., Nagamatsu, M., Ueo, H., and Akiyoshi, T. Enhanced induction of lymphokine-activated killer activity after lentinan administration in patients with gastric carcinoma. Int.J.Immunopharmacol. 1992;14(4):535-539.

[154] Gao, Y., Zhou, S., Jiang, W., Huang, M., and Dai, X. Effects of ganopoly (a Ganoderma lucidum polysaccharide extract) on the immune functions in advanced-stage cancer patients. Immunol.Invest 2003;32(3):201-215.

[155] Schultze, J. L., Stettin, A., and Berg, P. A. Demonstration of specifically sensitised lymphocytes in patients treated with an aqueous mistletoe extract (Viscum album L.). Klin.Wochenschr. 6-18-1991;69(9):397-403.

[156] Fidan I, Ozkan S, Gurbuz I, Yesilyurt E, Erdal B, Yolbakan S, Imir T. The efficiency of Viscum album ssp. album and Hypericum perforatum on human immune cells in vitro. Immunopharmacol Immunotoxicol. 2008;30(3):519-28.

[157] Terakawa, N., Matsui, Y., Satoi, S., Yanagimoto, H., Takahashi, K., Yamamoto, T., Yamao, J., Takai, S., Kwon, A. H., and Kamiyama, Y. Immunological effect of active hexose correlated compound (AHCC) in healthy volunteers: a double-blind, placebo-controlled trial. Nutr.Cancer 2008;60(5):643-651.

[158] Dellinger, EP, Babineau, TJ, and Bleicher, P. Effect of PGG-glucan on the rate of serious postoperative infection or death observed after high-risk gastrointestinal operations. Arch Surg 1999;1999(134):977-983.

[159] Lamm, S., Sheng, Y., and Pero, R. W. Persistent response to pneumococcal vaccine in individuals supplemented with a novel water soluble extract of Uncaria tomentosa, C-Med-100. Phytomedicine 2001;8(4):267-274.